Men's Fitness magazine

YOUR COMPLETE TRANSFORMATION GUIDE

12 WEEK BODY PLAN

by Nick Mitchell and Joe Warner

Art Editor Richard Davis
Additional design Jo Gurney
Managing Editor Chris Miller
Subeditors Gareth Beach, Jo Williams
Art Director Donovan Walker
Photography Tom Miles, Duncan Nicholls,
Glen Burrows, Danny Bird, Shutterstock

MAGBOOK

Group Publisher **Russell Blackman**
Group Managing Director **Ian Westwood**
Digital Production Manager **Nicky Baker**
International Business Development
Director **Dharmesh Mistry**
Operations Director **Robin Ryan**
Managing Director of Advertising
Julian Lloyd-Evans
Newstrade Director **David Barker**
Commercial & Retail Director **Martin Belson**
Chief Operating Officer/
Chief Financial Officer **Brett Reynolds**
Group Finance Director **Ian Leggett**
Chief Executive Officer **James Tye**
Chairman **Felix Dennis**

The 'MagBook' brand is a trademark of Dennis Publishing Ltd,
30 Cleveland Street, London W1T 4JD.
Company registered in England.
All material © Dennis Publishing Ltd, licensed by Felden 2012,
and may not be reproduced in whole or part without the
consent of the publishers. Printed in China.

12-WEEK BODY PLAN ISBN **1-78106-057-6**
To license this product please contact Nicole Adams on
+44 (0) 20 7907 6134 or nicole_adams@dennis.co.uk

Advertising
Katie Wood katie_wood@dennis.co.uk
Matt Wakefield matt_wakefield@dennis.co.uk

To subscribe to *Men's Fitness* magazine,
call **0844 844 0081** or go to **mensfitness.co.uk**

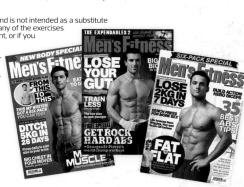

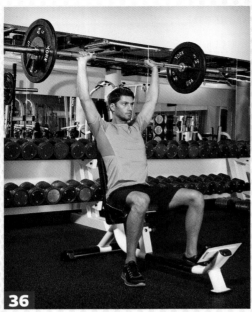

36

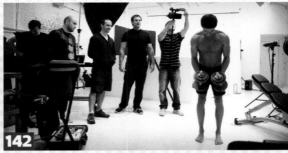

142

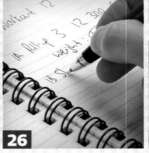

26

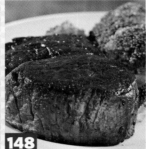

148

CONTENTS

ABOUT THIS BOOK   8
Foreword by Charles Poliquin •
About the book • About the authors

GETTING STARTED   14
Cover model muscle • How to do the challenge •
Workout planner • Tracking your progress •
Q&A • How muscles work • Glossary

MICROCYCLE 1 – WORKOUTS 1-8   36
Upper body • Lower body

MICROCYCLE 2 – WORKOUTS 9-17   44
Back and shoulders • Legs • Chest and arms

MICROCYCLE 3 – WORKOUTS 18-20   58
Back and shoulders • Legs • Chest and arms

MICROCYCLE 4 – WORKOUTS 21-29   70
Back and shoulders • Legs • Chest and arms

MICROCYCLE 5 – WORKOUTS 30-38   82
Back and shoulders • Legs • Chest and arms

MICROCYCLE 6 – WORKOUTS 39-41   98
Back and shoulders • Legs • Chest and arms

MICROCYCLE 7 – WORKOUTS 42-44   112
Back and shoulders • Legs • Chest and arms

MICROCYCLE 8 – WORKOUTS 45-46   124
Legs and arms • Chest, back and shoulders

ABS AND FAT LOSS   134
Six-pack science • Abs exercises •
High-intensity interval training • Fasted walking

FINISHING TOUCHES   142
Perfecting your cover model look

NUTRITION   148
Food rules • Q&A • Seven-day meal plan

SUPPLEMENTS   158
Why supplements work • Muscle • Fat loss • Health

TRAINING DIARY   168
Log every workout

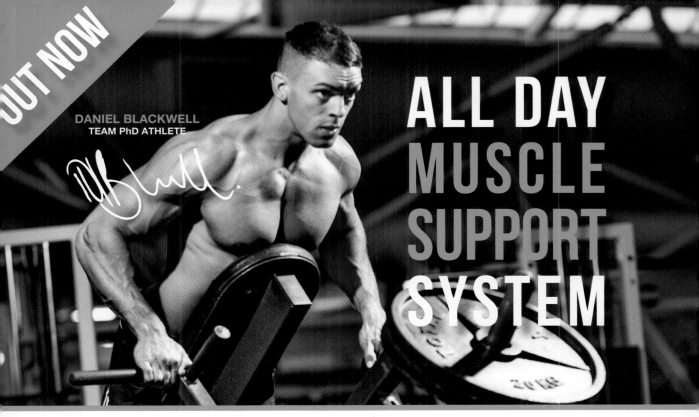

OUT NOW

DANIEL BLACKWELL
TEAM PhD ATHLETE

ALL DAY MUSCLE SUPPORT SYSTEM

NEW PHARMA PRO-3 PROTEIN BLEND

Pharma Pro-3™ is a professional protein blend made with Whey Protein, Milk Protein Isolate and Peptide Bonded L-Glutamine. It is a high protein dietary supplement designed to support the growth and maintenance of lean muscle. Combining effective amounts of Whey Protein Concentrate, Milk Protein Isolate (Containing approximately 80% Casein) and Peptide Bonded L-Glutamine (Derived from Hydrolysed Wheat Protein Isolate), Pharma Pro-3 is one of PhD Nutrition's most versatile high protein products and can be used at all times throughout the day to support intense training. A great tasting high protein shake, Pharma Pro-3 has been designed to supplement the diet and training of all athletes, from the elite to the beginner.

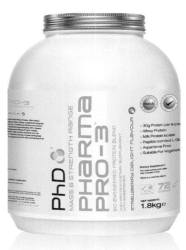

+ WHEY PROTEIN   + MILK PROTEIN ISOLATE

+ PEPTIDE BONDED L-GLUTAMINE   + ASPARTAME FREE

+ HIGH IN NATURALLY OCCURRING BCAA'S   + AVAILABLE IN 4 GREAT TASTING FLAVOURS

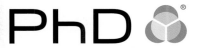 INNOVATION FOR THE MODERN ATHLETE

www.phd-supplements.com   Find us on:

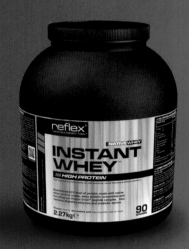

IT'S ALL IN THE
NUMBERS

Instant Whey™

Instant Whey™ with native whey is set to change the face of sports nutrition.

We partnered with one of the world's newest, most sophisticated and environmentally sound dairies to bring you native whey protein isolate extracted directly from fresh skimmed milk. It is this superior process that is carried out at low temperature via complex ultra and membrane filtration that captures virtually every single highly valuable biologically active protein fraction in its native form.

As a result it contains up to 166% more bioavailable cystine (two cysteine molecules linked by a disulphide bridge) and up to 16% more L-leucine than other forms of whey protein.

Add to this, the fantastic flavours, guaranteed protein levels and Full Money Back Guarantee and you can start to understand why it is the first choice for so many people.

80% protein

upto **16%** more L-leucine

upto **166%** more bioavailable cystine

www.reflex-nutrition.com

 Reflex Nutrition Ltd

 @ReflexNutrition

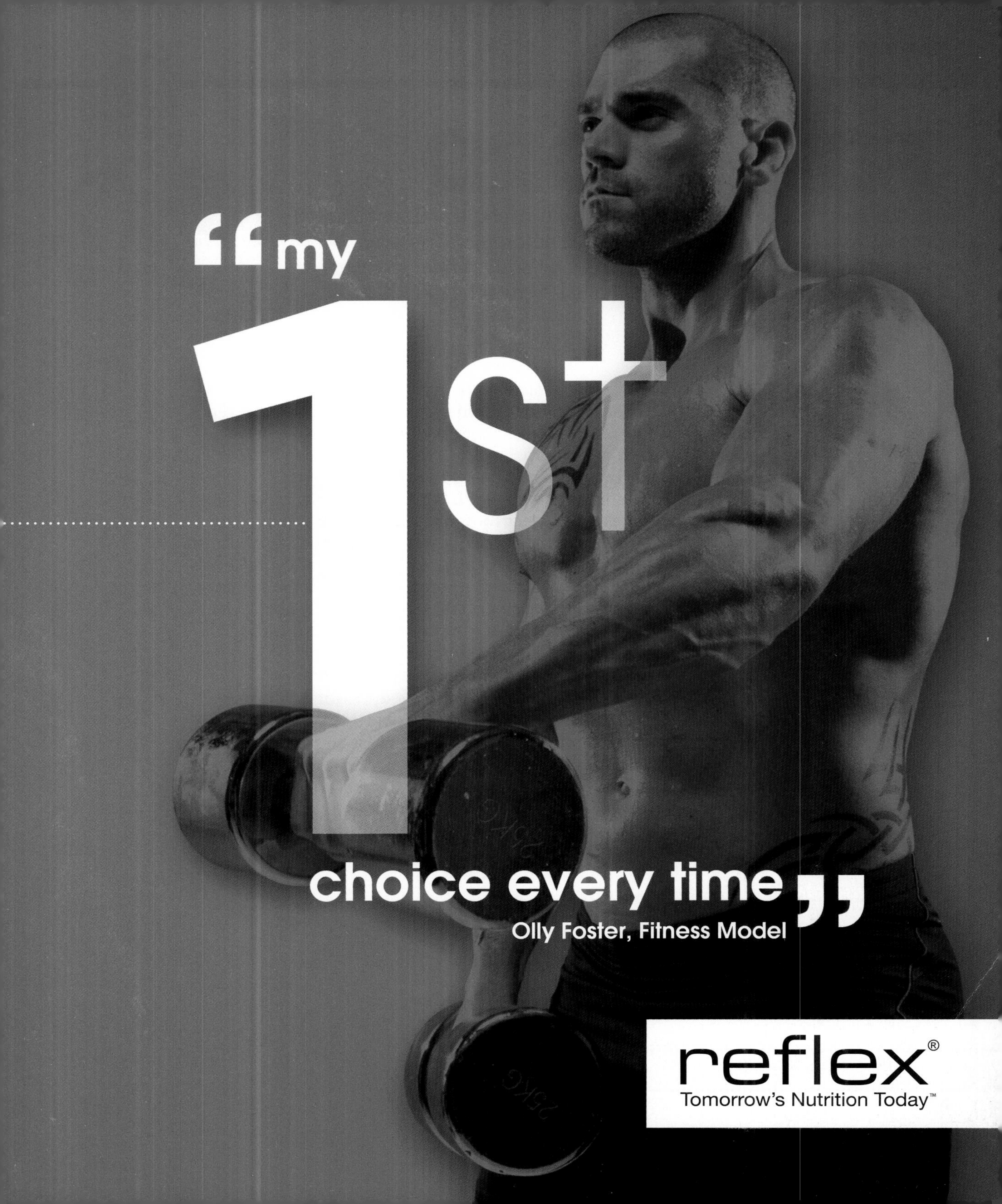

"my 1st
choice every time"
Olly Foster, Fitness Model
reflex®
Tomorrow's Nutrition Today™

FOREWORD

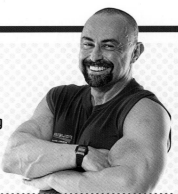

by Charles Poliquin, the world-renowned strength and conditioning coach, who has trained Olympians in 12 different sports, world record holders in ten different sports, and professional athletes in the NBA, NFL, NHL, MLB and English Premier League

I have known Nick Mitchell for more than five years, and during that time he has been responsible for many phenomenal transformations, helping people get the bodies they coveted. But it is his work with Joe Warner that has cemented his position as not only the leading body composition expert in Europe but also one of the best in the world.

I first met Joe when I started contributing to *Men's Fitness* magazine as its muscle expert. I even trained Joe once for a magazine feature. Although he tried hard, nothing I saw Joe do that day suggested he was capable of building enough muscle while burning enough fat to get on the cover of *Men's Fitness*. Indeed, I'd go as far as to say that his performance was as dynamic as that of a teddy bear on Valium, with a physique that would have only got him a game in a primary school football match if they were short of a goalpost.

However, Nick has demonstrated that a smart, well-planned training programme and nutrition plan can lead to a remarkable change in the way you look without a shirt on. The exercise and diet framework are only half the battle, of course. You could learn Nick's programme inside out, but it won't have any effect unless you execute it with the same focus, determination and desire that Joe did.

And that's the key to you getting the same results as Joe. You need to follow every single one of Nick's instructions as if your life depended upon it. Attack this programme with a full heart and clear eyes and you will be astonished by what you achieve.

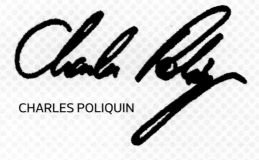

CHARLES POLIQUIN

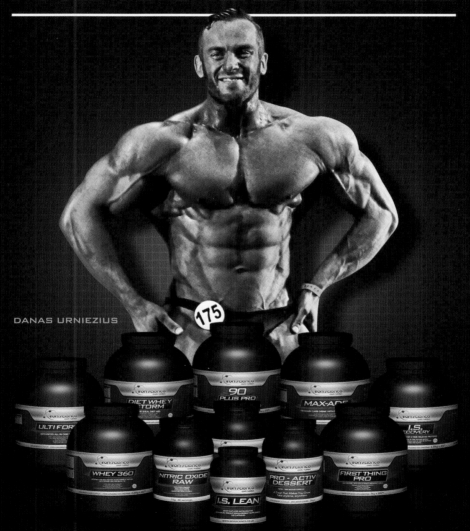

ABOUT THE BOOK

Here's why this book is the only guide you will ever need to getting the physique you have always wanted

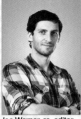

Joe Warner, co-editor

The fitness industry is filled with personal trainers and authors who claim that they can dramatically change the way you look with minimum fuss, effort or expense. This book is a bit different. That's because genuine transformations – where your body changes so rapidly and so significantly that friends, family and colleagues can't help but comment on the size of your biceps or try to poke at your shrinking belly to see how hard your abs are – require hard training with utter dedication and commitment to building a body you have always wanted.

Trust me, I know. That's because I trained under the guidance of Nick Mitchell to discover how radically I could transform my physique in just 12 weeks with the right training and nutrition plan.

The complete guide

This book contains the complete programme that I followed for 12 weeks, detailing every single workout and when to do it. As well as the nutrition plan Nick created for me to stick to, there's a comprehensive overview of how you can eat better and smarter for a stronger, leaner body. It also includes the only guide to building a six-pack you'll need, featuring the only types of cardio training you should do to burn belly fat. And there's a complete guide to the best supplements available to support muscle-building, fat-burning and general health.

So if you have ever wanted to build a big, strong and lean body this is the book for you. And the beauty is that, if you follow this programme to the letter, you are going to achieve this physique in just 12 weeks. So start now. Why would you wait?

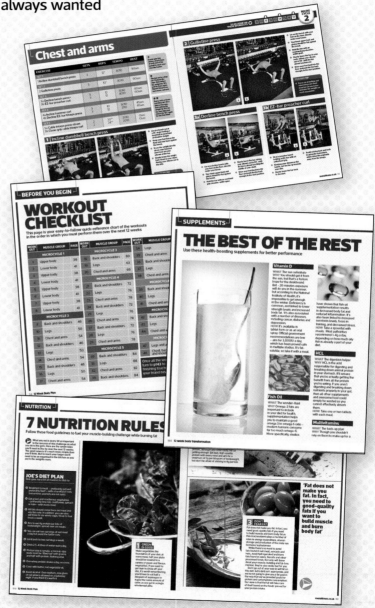

THE AUTHORS

The two men behind this book collaborated to transform a beer-swilling journalist into a cover model in 12 weeks. Here's what makes them tick

About Nick Mitchell

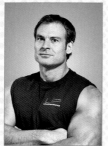

Nick is the founder of Ultimate Performance (upfitness.co.uk), the UK's foremost personal training business, and is widely recognised as one of the world's leading personal trainers and body composition experts. A former competitive strength and physique athlete, Nick has worked with an array of professional athletes, bodybuilders, movie and pop stars, but he is best known for his ability to radically change a client's physique in record time.

The fitness world knows that working with Nick is never easy, but always effective. Everything he does is rooted in a rigorous methodology, so that he can predict for his clients the exact changes their bodies will make, instilling confidence and transparency into a process that in the past has too often been clouded by haphazard guesswork. Nothing is left to chance, with Nick ensuring

'Nick Mitchell has become one of the most sought-after experts in fitness'

that every single area that could have an impact on his clients' performance and physical well-being is first audited and then managed and demystified for maximum results.

Nick has become one of the most sought-after experts in the fitness world and is known as the man who can get anyone 'cover model ready'. Nick's empowering teaching style motivates his clients to reach beyond their self-imposed limitations and achieve results that they never thought possible.
Follow Nick on Twitter @UPFitness

About Joe Warner

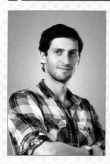

Joe is the deputy editor of *Men's Fitness* magazine. He has never been a strength and physique athlete and his greatest achievements in the sporting arena are representing the county of Essex at chess at under-nine and under-11 level (losing every match) and running four marathons with a distinctly average PB of 3hr 29min 47sec.

He has, however, been on the cover of *Men's Fitness* magazine after completing a 12-week training programme devised and overseen by Nick Mitchell. He approached Nick after spending most of his 20s chasing a better physique but never really getting anywhere, despite spending hours in the gym and running on the road.

It turned out everything he thought he knew about building muscle and burning fat was wrong. Luckily Nick was happy to help turn the 30-year-old beer-drinking, biscuit-scoffing journalist into a genuine cover model, complete with a six-pack. He genuinely

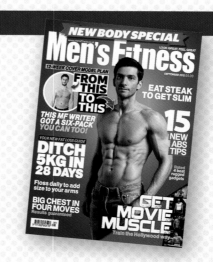

believes that if he can do it, so can you, which is why he and Nick have written this book.
Follow Joe on Twitter @JoeWarnerMF

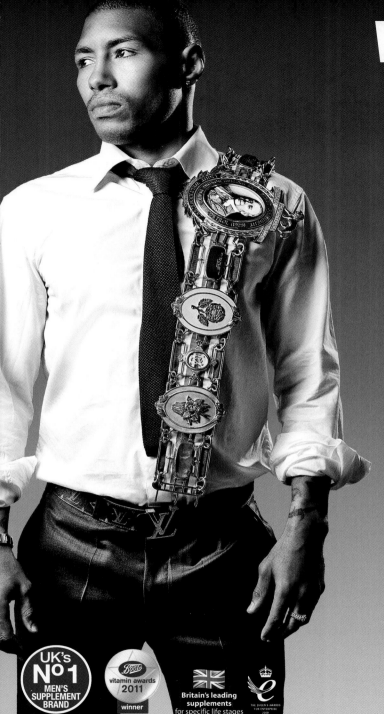
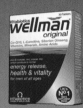 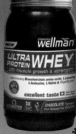
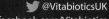

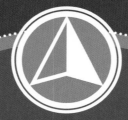

BEFORE YOU BEGIN

Read this chapter to understand how this training programme works and what you need to do before beginning your journey to a brand new body

BRAND NEW YOU

Here's how you are going to get bigger, stronger and leaner

This first chapter sets the scene for the next 12 weeks, explaining in detail everything you need to know before beginning my 12-week programme that builds muscle and burns fat to transform your physique into the one you have always wanted. It's essential that you read the following pages before you start training to understand exactly how it will work so you'll be armed with everything you need to attack your new training plan and diet with focus, determination and desire.

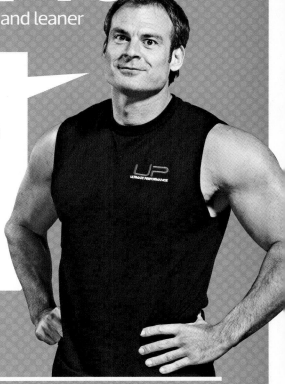

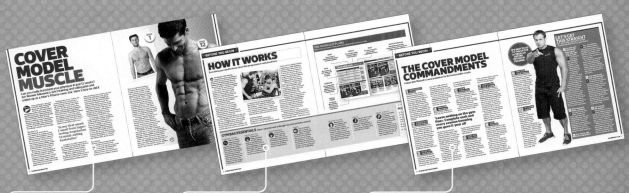

P16 Read how Joe Warner transformed his body in 12 weeks and how he dealt with the ups, downs and demands of Nick Mitchell's arduous programme

P22 All the information you need to follow this training plan, from an explanation of the sessions to what you need to put in your gym bag

P28 Coach Mitchell sets out the rules you must follow if you want his programme to produce impressive results – and answers the vital questions

COVER MODEL MUSCLE

Can you really transform your physique in just 12 weeks? Joe Warner followed a strict training and eating plan and ended up as a *Men's Fitness* cover star. Here's how he did it

I have never had a six-pack in my life. Well, technically I have, but until recently I'd never seen it because it was hidden under a thick layer of fat. I wouldn't mind, but I spent most of my 20s chasing a better physique. Despite hours in the gym and lots of long-distance running, I wasn't particularly strong or muscular and I constantly carried a little belly, even when I was running a sub-3hr 30min marathon. Something, I realised, had to change.

The big 3-0

What changed, it turned out, was hitting 30. A sudden, painful awareness that I might live my life without ever seeing the outline of my abdominals convinced me to find out what I was doing wrong and seek professional help. Could a beer-drinking, biscuit-scoffing journalist build a body worthy of a *Men's Fitness* cover model?

To find out, I enlisted the help of Nick Mitchell, founder of Ultimate Performance Fitness with two personal training gyms in London (upfitness.co.uk), who is one of the most highly sought-after body composition experts in the country. Initial diagnosis: not good.

'You have the classic "skinny-fat" ectomorphic body, meaning you have not much muscle but a lot of fat, specifically on your belly,' Nick told me. 'It's the result of genetics, a high-carb, low-protein vegetarian diet, a demanding job, high stress levels and years of endurance training. We need to lose a lot of fat, while also adding a significant amount of new lean tissue to your slow-twitch, marathon-running muscles. It's not mission impossible, but it's close.'

'In my first week I went from lager-loving vegetarian to meat-eating teetotaller'

Luckily for me, Nick is always up for a challenge. He agreed to oversee my training and diet for 12 weeks on two conditions: that I started eating meat and gave up alcohol.

The first wasn't a tough sell. Despite not eating mammals, fish or fowl for the past 21 years, I'd been contemplating starting again for a while, mainly because I can't cook and was fed up eating the same things every day. I was also struggling to consume enough protein and other vital nutrients found in meat. The prospect that going carnivore would help my mission was the final straw. As it turns out meat is delicious, and I instantly felt better and had more energy. I'm not saying you *have* to eat meat to change your body – but it certainly worked for me.

As for booze, I knew it would be tough, but I tried to think of hopping on the wagon as a short-term sacrifice for long-term gain. In my first week with Nick I went from lager-loving vegetarian to meat-eating teetotaller. Not just going cold turkey, but actually starting to eat it. My diet was built around lean protein and lots of vegetables and was, fortunately for a man of my culinary skills, pretty simple.

Fat attack

My first session began with Nick measuring my body fat using callipers to work out where my body likes to store fat. This helped him build up a picture of what my hormones were doing, and which supplements I needed to balance

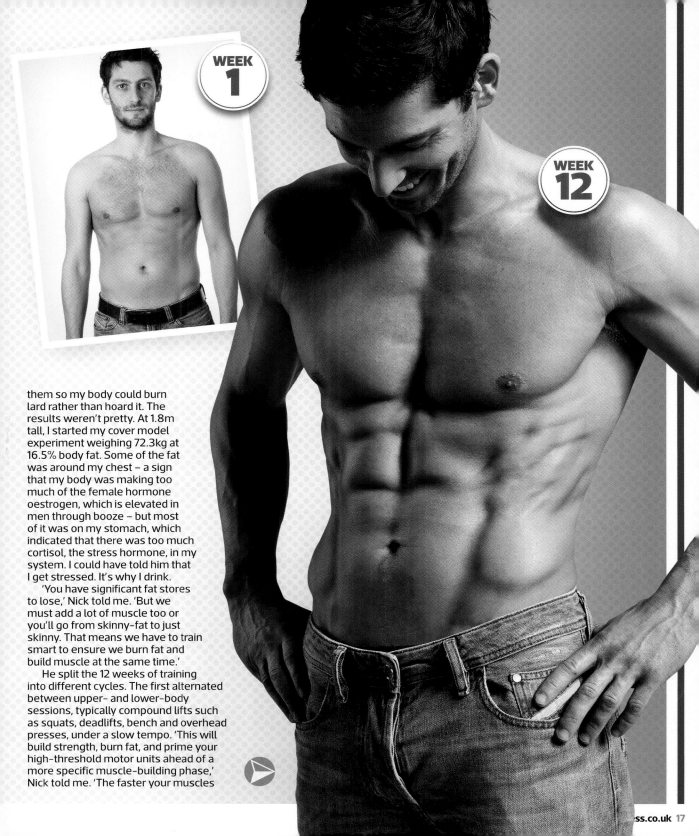

WEEK 1

WEEK 12

them so my body could burn lard rather than hoard it. The results weren't pretty. At 1.8m tall, I started my cover model experiment weighing 72.3kg at 16.5% body fat. Some of the fat was around my chest – a sign that my body was making too much of the female hormone oestrogen, which is elevated in men through booze – but most of it was on my stomach, which indicated that there was too much cortisol, the stress hormone, in my system. I could have told him that I get stressed. It's why I drink.

'You have significant fat stores to lose,' Nick told me. 'But we must add a lot of muscle too or you'll go from skinny-fat to just skinny. That means we have to train smart to ensure we burn fat and build muscle at the same time.'

He split the 12 weeks of training into different cycles. The first alternated between upper- and lower-body sessions, typically compound lifts such as squats, deadlifts, bench and overhead presses, under a slow tempo. 'This will build strength, burn fat, and prime your high-threshold motor units ahead of a more specific muscle-building phase,' Nick told me. 'The faster your muscles learn to contract, the harder we can push them later to pack on muscle.'

Nick also emphasised that what I consumed before, during and after my sessions would be hugely influential in creating the conditions to make maximum changes. He put me on a pre-workout drink full of caffeine and beta-alanine, a type of amino acid. It really worked, helping me focus and improving blood flow into my muscles. It also made my face and hands tingle – a sensation that sometimes extended as far as my testicles, which was something of an unadvertised bonus.

I also popped three branched-chain amino acid (BCAA) pills after every set. These prevent muscle breakdown while promoting protein synthesis. The result is bigger, stronger muscles, so necking 40 pills per workout is well worth the trouble.

March of progress

After two full weeks of brutal workouts, training Monday, Wednesday and Friday lunchtimes and Saturday mornings, I was already seeing results. The exercises stayed the same, but the weights moved up every session and in two weeks I dropped my body

'After two weeks of brutal workouts I was already seeing results'

fat percentage from 16.5% to 12.8% while adding a couple of kilograms of lean muscle. It was a good start (so good that it prompted disbelieving comments on UP's Facebook page) but only convinced Nick to push harder.

'A common mistake when trying to build muscle is to lift the same weight every workout,' he said. 'If you don't make your muscles do something they've not done before they have no incentive to grow.'

The upper-body sessions were hard, but not as tough as the legs sessions, mainly because I had very weak legs. Great for running long distances, useless at shifting heavy barbells. Nick started calling me Ostrich, not just because my

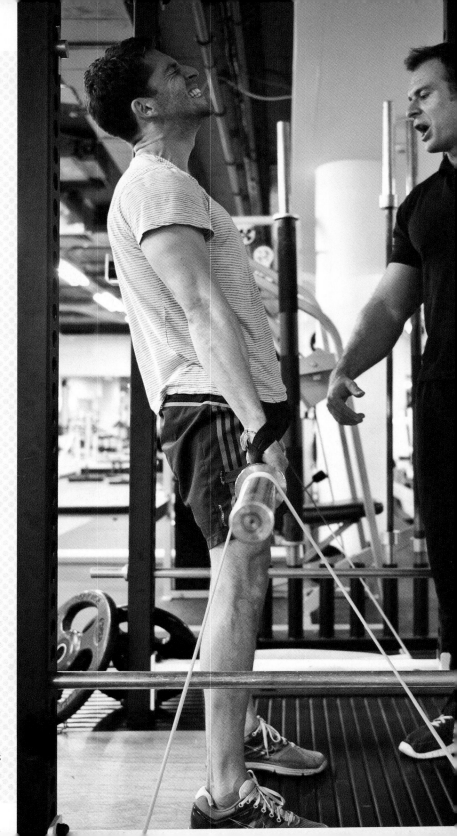

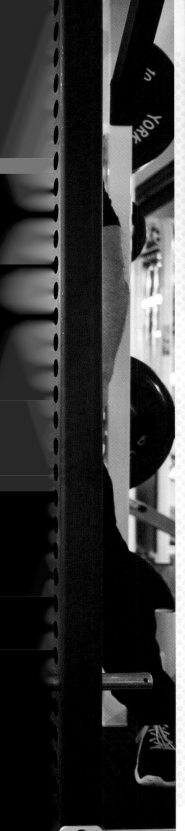

Joe Warner
VITAL STATISTICS

Starting weight	72.3kg
End weight	74.3kg
Starting body-fat percentage	16.5%
End body-fat percentage	5.5%
Fat lost	8kg
Muscle gained	10kg
Total workouts	48
Most eggs eaten in 24 hours	11
Invitations to the pub turned down	14
T-shirts that no longer fit	All of them

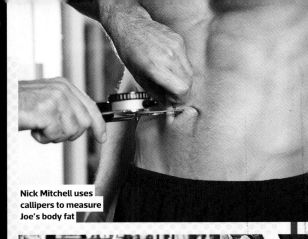

Nick Mitchell uses callipers to measure Joe's body fat

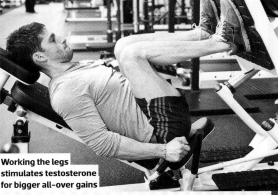

Working the legs stimulates testosterone for bigger all-over gains

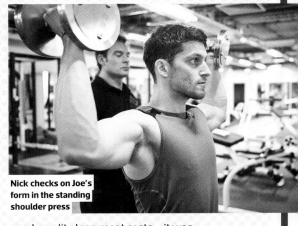

Nick checks on Joe's form in the standing shoulder press

legs were so skinny, but because I'd been sticking my head in the sand about legs training to focus solely on my 'mirror' muscles – chest, arms and shoulders.

'Your legs are your biggest muscles, so you can lift heavier weights to release more testosterone and growth hormones that will instruct your body to build muscle and burn your love handles,' he told me. Unfortunately, they are also the muscles most prone to filling with lactic acid and leaving me squirming on the floor. Still, the balanced approach was getting results.

Man vs Food

Of course, as we often emphasise in *Men's Fitness*, what you do in the gym is only half the challenge. The other is eating the right foods at the right time to fuel your progress. The good news for my cover model body was that Nick's preferred fat-trimming, muscle-building diet is ridiculously simple to understand. The bad news? It's hard to follow – unless you're organised.

I started batch-cooking lean mince with vegetables, which I had for dinner and took to work for lunch. Packets of cooked chicken replaced crisps in my shopping basket. Eating out wasn't too bad: most places do steak or chicken and will let you swap carb-heavy foods for extra vegetables. All you have to do is ask, then try not to pinch anyone's chips.

Not only was following this diet expensive – as a newly converted carnivore I couldn't believe how much

good-quality lean meat costs – it was also dull. Seriously dull. Eating became a bit of a chore. I stopped looking forward to meal times, and when they came around I could barely look at the slices of beef stacked up on my plate. But as Nick kept reminding me, I was eating for my muscles, not my taste buds.

'Forgetting' to eat wasn't an option. In Nick's own words, 'Skipping a meal is worse than skipping a workout.

If you do that you're wasting your own time and, even worse, you're wasting mine.' So I kept munching dutifully away on all the protein-packed meat and nutrient-rich veg.

Time to split
By week three Nick had changed up my training to a three-way body part split, training back and shoulders in one session, then legs, then chest and arms. But every session was different, thanks to Nick's constant tinkering with sets, reps, tempo, rest and even exercise selection. Since my muscles were always being asked to do something new, they had no option but to keep growing.

'It's tempting to do three sets of eight reps for every exercise in every session,' said Nick. 'But after a few weeks your muscles know exactly what's in store and can cope with the load. Even increasing the weight isn't always enough to keep them growing. You have to tweak every variable to keep progressing. You should always be outside your comfort zone.'

No problem there. I never rested for more than about 90 seconds between sets or exercises. This intensity sent my heart-rate soaring, as well as increasing lactic acid levels to help torch fat.

'To build muscle and burn fat you need to work out hard and fast because testosterone, the muscle-building hormone, peaks 45 to 60 minutes into

For quick results, bodyweight isn't always enough

a workout,' Nick told me. 'Then it falls away rapidly and cortisol levels rise. This stress hormone not only prevents your body from burning fat, it actually instructs it to store more.'

Carb alarm
In week six I finally got a treat. For the first month and a half of the cover model plan I avoided all carbs except vegetables. But now I was getting leaner – my body fat crept close to 10% – Nick reintroduced carbs to my diet to keep my muscles fuelled, starting in my post-workout shake and increasing gradually as I shed more fat. I was also allowed a bowl of porridge before bed on the days I trained.

The carb infusion didn't do much for my taste buds but it did help my muscles and give me more energy in the gym. This came in handy when Nick decided to shake things up again by making me do three or even four different exercises back to back without

Tracking Joe's progress
TAKING SHAPE

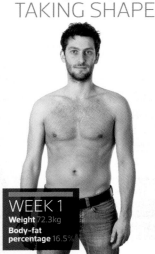

WEEK 1
Weight 72.3kg
Body-fat percentage 16.5%

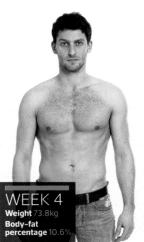

WEEK 4
Weight 73.8kg
Body-fat percentage 10.6%

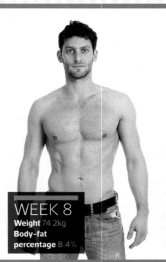

WEEK 8
Weight 74.2kg
Body-fat percentage 8.4%

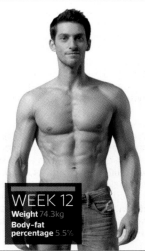

WEEK 12
Weight 74.3kg
Body-fat percentage 5.5%

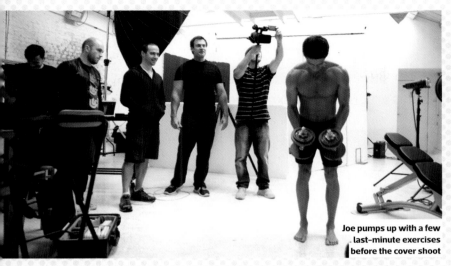

'I started doing a high-intensity interval sessions once a week to shift the stubborn fat on my belly'

Joe pumps up with a few last-minute exercises before the cover shoot

rest. Typically this would be one big compound move followed by isolation, or single-joint, lifts.

'To achieve maximum stimulation so the muscle fibres grow back bigger, isolation movements are the way to go,' Nick said. 'They are less taxing on your nervous system than compound lifts so you can go to town with the volume you lift in a session to stimulate your muscles.' I also did a lot of drop sets, which is when you do a move to failure, then continue with a lighter weight. Working the muscles to complete fatigue is effective, but it's not pleasant. The burn it creates made me hop on the spot, clench my fists and invent some fairly colourful swearword combos.

My shoulders, arms and legs were bigger and my chest was more defined, but the six-pack was still nowhere to be seen. So I started doing a high-intensity interval session once a week to shift the fat stubbornly sticking to my belly, in a bid to turn my two-pack into the full half-dozen that cover models need to pay the bills.

Core concerns
With a fortnight to go, the programme was undeniably working. My body fat levels were falling each week while I was still getting heavier, proof that I was packing on muscle. But I couldn't help worrying that my abs were still refusing to blossom into a full six-pack. I'd always believed that doing lots of big lifts, especially squats

and shoulder presses, was enough to get rock-solid abs, but it's not.

'The abs are like any other muscle group – they need to be targeted directly,' Nick told me. 'You have poor abs, in that they aren't very thick. That's genetics, so we need to work even harder over the final two weeks to bring them out as much as possible.'

From that day forward, every other workout included some agonising abs work. Barbell roll-outs, done super-slow, were the worst. Hanging legs raises and weighted crunches aren't much fun either, but they're effective at sculpting a six-pack, as long as you've shifted the fat on top of them first.

With my final session in the bag – a horrible hour of tri-sets and drop sets to flush as much blood into my muscles while also stripping their cells of any glucose to make me look as lean as possible - Nick gave me one final order:

to get a spray tan. 'You'll look 10-20% better with a tan because it'll highlight your new muscles and make them look leaner,' he promised me. In an effort not to look like a *Hollyoaks* extra I tried to get the best available, going to celebrity tanner James Read at the Agua Spa at London's Sanderson hotel. I emerged after 20 minutes looking as if I'd spent two weeks in the Caribbean, much to the amusement of the rest of the office.

Take cover
The day before the shoot Nick put me through a final body fat assessment, with results that were little short of unbelievable. In 12 weeks I'd lost 8kg of fat and added 10kg of lean muscle. I'm now stronger, leaner and heavier than I've ever been. And for the first time in my life I am the owner of a six-pack.

It took hard work and discipline, but by giving your all every time you step into your gym and by eating the right foods at the right time you *can* transform your body into the one you've always wanted. You might not make it on to the cover of *MF*, but who knows? If I can do it, anyone can.

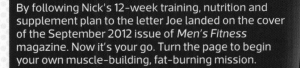

NOW IT'S YOUR TURN ➢

By following Nick's 12-week training, nutrition and supplement plan to the letter Joe landed on the cover of the September 2012 issue of *Men's Fitness* magazine. Now it's your go. Turn the page to begin your own muscle-building, fat-burning mission.

For the video of Joe's cover model challenge go to **mensfitness.co.uk/links/covermodeljoe**

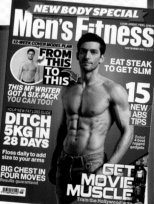

HOW IT WORKS

Everything you need to know about this programme is explained here

 The beauty of this training programme is that everything is laid out for you for the next 12 weeks. It's the exact workout plan that Joe followed to get into shape to be on the cover of *Men's Fitness* magazine.

The entire 12-week plan is called a mesocycle. This mesocycle is broken down into eight smaller phases or microcycles, each of which has a specific aim that will prepare you for the following cycle, while also working towards the overall objective: building you a brand new body.

Each microcycle includes two or three different workouts, so to make the programme easy to follow, each cycle has its own chapter containing all the workouts you do in that particular microcycle before moving on to the next one.

The plan has been devised in this way because building muscle is not a linear process. Doing the same exercise with the same weight for the same number of sets and reps each session may result in a few quick gains, but these will quickly plateau as your muscles become

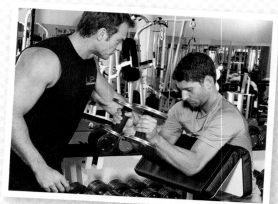

accustomed to the demands placed upon them. Only regularly shaking up the variables – such as the moves your perform, the weight you use and the sets and reps you complete – will ensure you continue to build new muscle tissue while burning away unwanted fat stores.

Getting started

Before you begin the training programme, read this chapter to familiarise yourself with what lies

ahead. Then read the nutrition chapter, beginning on p148, and the supplements chapter on p158. Building a better body is about what you do in the kitchen as much as it is what you do in the gym, so follow the food rules detailed to give your body the nutrients it needs to fuel your muscle-building and fat-loss mission.

With your nutrition plan in place, you are ready to start. You will be hitting the gym four times a week. Joe trained on Monday, Wednesday and Friday lunchtimes and Saturday mornings. This fitted in with his work schedule and gave him time to recover, which is the key to building muscle and burning fat. Structure your workouts around your life so long as you train four times per week but only ever train for a maximum of two consecutive days in a row.

All the exercises, sets, reps, tempo and rest periods are clearly detailed, so pack your gym bag with what you need – including this book – and away you go.

GYM BAG ESSENTIALS Here's what Joe took to the gym for each and every session

TRAINING DIARY
 This is crucial to staying on track. Make sure you spend five or ten minutes before training writing down all the information you need for that session so you'll know exactly what you need to do and don't waste any training time. You can use any notebook or the version in this book (see p168).

WATER BOTTLE
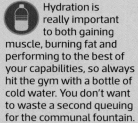 Hydration is really important to both gaining muscle, burning fat and performing to the best of your capabilities, so always hit the gym with a bottle of cold water. You don't want to waste a second queuing for the communal fountain.

SUPPLEMENTS
Joe took three BCAA capsules after every set to prevent muscle tissue breakdown and promote new muscle growth (see p158 for our complete guide to supplements).

TOWEL
You are going to get to sweaty, so have a small gym towel with you to wipe down kit and equipment after you use it. It's just good manners. You'll also need to it to dry you hands so your grip is as strong as it needs to be for moves such as chin-ups and deadlifts.

THE WORKOUT PLANS
Here's how to do each of the workouts and what the key terms mean

REPS
The number of repetitions of the move you must complete

TEMPO
The speed at which you must perform each repetition

REST
The time in seconds you rest after completing the move

NAVIGATION BAR
This details which of the workout microcycles you are on and the workouts within it

SETS
The number of sets of the move you must complete

EXERCISE
The names of the moves you are going to do in the order they need to be performed

VISUAL GUIDE
Joe Warner demonstrates the start and end position of each move

FORM
Clear and detailed written descriptions of how to perform each move

TRAINER TIPS
These are Nick Mitchell's expert tips to bear in mind when doing this exercise

Chest and arms

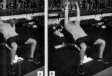

PROTEIN SHAKE
What you eat immediately after your session is crucial. Prepare a whey-packed protein shake so it's ready for you as soon as you've completed your final rep to give your muscles the nutrients they need to grow back bigger and stronger.

CHALK
Joe had never used chalk before but found it really useful for squeezing out a few extra – and important – reps when his grip would have otherwise failed.

WRIST STRAPS
These are helpful for pulling movements such as deadlifts and chin-ups. Using these straps means your grip is secured, meaning you can focus on working the target muscle groups. You may not need them on low-rep sets, but they are ideal for sets of more than five reps.

Before you begin

✔ Read this chapter throughly

✔ Read the chapters on nutrition (p148) and supplements (p158)

✔ Buy your gym bag essentials

✔ Start training!

WORKOUT CHECKLIST

This page is your easy-to-follow quick-reference chart of the workouts in the order in which you must perform them over the next 12 weeks

WORK OUT	MUSCLE GROUP	PAGE	WORK OUT	MUSCLE GROUP	PAGE	WORK OUT	MUSCLE GROUP	PAGE
MICROCYCLE 1			**MICROCYCLE 3**			34	Legs	88
1	Upper body	38	18	Back and shoulders	60	35	Chest and arms	92
2	Lower body	41	19	Legs	63	36	Back and shoulders	84
3	Upper body	38	20	Chest and arms	66	37	Legs	88
4	Lower body	41	**MICROCYCLE 4**			38	Chest and arms	92
5	Upper body	38	21	Back and shoulders	72	**MICROCYCLE 6**		
6	Lower body	41	22	Legs	76	39	Back and shoulders	100
7	Upper body	38	23	Chest and arms	78	40	Legs	104
8	Lower body	41	24	Back and shoulders	72	41	Chest and arms	108
MICROCYCLE 2			25	Legs	76	**MICROCYCLE 7**		
9	Back and shoulders	46	26	Chest and arms	78	42	Back and shoulders	114
10	Legs	50	27	Back and shoulders	72	43	Legs	118
11	Chest and arms	54	28	Legs	76	44	Chest and arms	120
12	Back and shoulders	46	29	Chest and arms	78	**MICROCYCLE 8**		
13	Legs	50	**MICROCYCLE 5**			47	Legs and arms	126
14	Chest and arms	54	30	Back and shoulders	84	46	Chest, back and shoulders	130
15	Back and shoulders	46	31	Legs	88			
16	Legs	50	32	Chest and arms	92			
17	Chest and arms	54	33	Back and shoulders	84			

Once all the workouts are done turn to **p142** to put the finishing touches to your brand new body

CLASS LEADING NUTRITION

PRO-6

The ultimate protein supplement designed to give you a full amino acid profile in a low fat and low carbohydate blend of multiple protein sources. Perfect for anyone looking to build, maintain or lose fat.

KREVOLUTION-X

This is Extreme Nutritions 1 of Kre-Alkalyn, an alkylated form of creatine which doesn't convert into the acidic creatinine in the stomach. Creatinine can cause stomach upset, water retention and kidney stress. We have blended this with Rhodiola Rosea, a herb popular in homeopathic medicine due to it being thought to boost the immune system, reduce stress, enhance endurance and it helps with the conversion of creatine into Adenosine Tri-Phosphate, the stuff your muscles use for energy whenever to contract a muscle, be it in the gym, in the ring or in the sack!

BUILD & RECOVER

The first post workout of it's kind. Extreme Nutrition were first to bring you a multi protein, multi carb post workout meal replacement/recovery drink with minerals, vitamins, HMB and Kre-Alkalyn. This product has undergone trials at Heriot Watt University in Edinburgh and was found to increase performance, strength and muscularity in double blind placebo tests.

RELOAD

A blend of natural herbs designed to boost male hormone production. In University studies the different ingredients in Reload have been shown to increase testosterone whilst lowering oestrogen! This product has been hugely popular amongst natural athletes, bodybuilders trying to return their endocrine systems to normal after taking steroids and older athletes who still want the hormone levels of a 20 something!

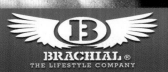

0845 365 3155
www.extremenutrition.co.uk

TRACKING YOUR PROGRESS

Stay on top of your transformation by taking the following steps

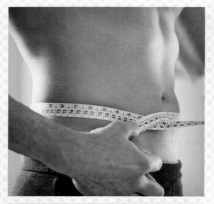

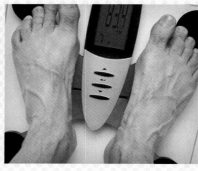

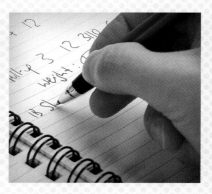

1 MEASURE YOURSELF

Your measurements are more important than your weight because this programme is about transforming your appearance, not about how much you weigh. Record your measurements with a tape measure around the following areas: shoulders, arms (with biceps flexed), chest (over the nipples) and stomach (around your belly button). You can also do hips, thighs and calves if you want a more complete picture. Then take measurements from the same sites every week or fortnight. It can be tricky to measure yourself accurately so get someone to help you. And don't use the start of the tape measure to assess circumferences, because it can go slack. Instead go 10cm over so that the tape is tight around the body part, and then subtract 10cm to get an accurate measurement.

2 WEIGH YOURSELF

Jump on the scales before you begin this programme to get a start weight that you can compare against each week or fortnight. Always use the same scales at the same time of day; it's best to do it first thing in the morning. It's easy to think you're not making progress if your weight is staying the same or even increasing. But weight is a bad indicator here: when you're building muscle and burning fat, the chances are that your weight won't go down. At the end of his programme Joe was the heaviest he'd ever been in his life, but also the leanest, which meant he looked totally different from when he started.

3 TAKE PHOTOS

What's important when tracking your progress is your body composition and the best way to monitor that is to take photos of yourself without a top on from the front, back and side. Do this before your first session, then every week or fortnight to get the best idea of how you are doing.

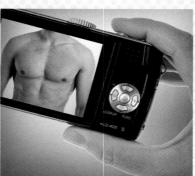

And always take these photos on the same day of the week and at the same time to get the most accurate report.

4 KEEP A DIARY

This book clearly details the exercises, sets, reps, tempo and rest for each and every workout you will do, but one thing you will need to keep track of is the weights you lift. Simply copy out that day's workout from this book in your diary before you go to the gym – or you can use the version we've provided (see p168) – and add in the weight you think you will need to select to hit your sets, rep and tempo target. After your first set put a tick next to the weight if you just about managed it, but if it was too light or heavy make an adjustment and note this down. After the session go back over your workout to make the best estimation of what you intend to lift next time.

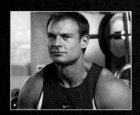
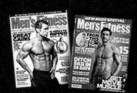
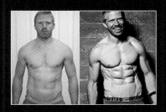
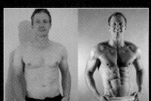
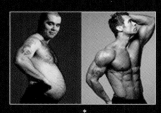
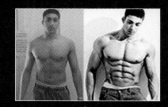

THE COVER MODEL COMMANDMENTS

Follow Nick Mitchell's crucial guidelines for the best possible results

1 CONSISTENCY IS KEY

The key to a successful physical transformation is the accumulated number of how many correct things you do every single day. Three good days of training hard and eating right followed by one bad day when you go off the rails does not equate to a net gain of two good days: the hormonal implications mean you will take some significant steps backwards. Every single day counts. Don't waste any of them.

2 INTENSITY IS EVERYTHING

You are only training in the gym for around four hours a week – that's nothing in the grand scheme of what you do each week. But these four hours are among the most important. Leave nothing on the gym floor. You should complete each and every session knowing you gave it your all. You should feel exhausted but ultimately delighted with your execution.

3 LISTEN TO YOUR BODY

For any training and diet regime to work properly, the more in tune you are with what your body is telling you the greater your chances of success. You need to be your own coach and be as objective and honest with yourself as possible. You can, and should, back off if you are physically exhausted – you'll do more harm than good – but you must also learn to distinguish between mental weakness and physical tiredness. Don't pull the wool over your own eyes.

4 MONITOR PROGRESS

Tracking your progress to help you stay motivated is

'Leave nothing on the gym floor. Complete each and every session knowing you gave it your all'

an absolute must to the success of this project. Take photos from the front, back and side before you start, and then every week or fortnight. You also need to track your weight-training sessions in a journal or you won't be able to ensure you're pushing for improved performance at each and every workout.

Try keeping a detailed food diary too. Unless you keep a written note of everything that goes in your mouth, it is remarkable how easy it is to either overeat or undereat, both of which are equally bad for your cover model aspirations.

5 KNOW YOUR GOAL

Joe succeeded in his quest because he had laser focus on what he wanted to achieve – to get on the cover of *Men's Fitness*. Work out your ultimate goal before you start and don't waver from it.

And be sure you are doing this for yourself, not to please anyone else. This is a very tough regime and for you to stick to it and succeed you must be motivated by the right intention.

6 SORT OUT YOUR LIFE

If you want the best body you've ever had then you need to make sacrifices. In particular, this means giving up nights in the pub, takeaways and burning the candle at both ends.

You need to prioritise what's more important to you: proving you can get the body you have always wanted or having a few pints after work on a Friday night?

7 LEAVE YOUR EGO AT HOME

Effective weight training is not about heaving as much weight as possible from point A to point B. What must be paramount in your mind while training is that the weights are mere tools and your job is to flex your muscles against those weights. This means you may have to reduce the weights you lift to ensure you stick to the required sets, reps, tempo and rest periods.

Remember: you're not lifting for your ego or to impress anyone. You are lifting for the most effective way to build new muscle.

8 STAY POSITIVE

Chances are it will be tough to stick to the entire 12-week programme without the odd setback. Work may get in the way, for example, and family and friends may demand more of your time.

When issues do pop up and threaten to derail your progress, take them in your stride. Don't let obstacles prevent you from training – you must find the time – or blow the diet. Stay strong and focused on the big picture.

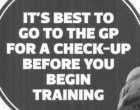

9 PRACTISE YOUR POSING

Flexing your muscles and practising your cover model poses aren't narcissistic, they're a necessity. They'll improve your mind-muscle connections, so you learn to contract a muscle group more quickly and with more force, which will result in you being able to better stimulate it when training. They'll allow you to get a better 'feel' for each muscle group, as well as improving definition once you start getting leaner.

10 GET SOME SLEEP

Sleep isn't a luxury, it's an absolute cornerstone of this programme. Poor-quality sleep will lead to lowered testosterone and growth hormone levels, as well as impaired blood-sugar management. Aim for eight to nine hours' uninterrupted sleep each and every night. Turn your bedroom into the Bat Cave: no lights on and no TV on standby, eliminate any noise with earplugs and try a supplement to promote sleep (see page 158).

LET'S GET THIS STRAIGHT

No-nonsense answers to the fundamental fitness questions

Q I've tried and failed to add muscle in the past. Why will it work now?

A If your efforts have been unsuccessful in the past, it has nothing to do with your body being resistant to exercise and everything to do with your approach. In other words, you haven't had a focused plan so you haven't set yourself realistic and achievable goals or eaten the right foods.
Anyone can make significant, positive changes to the way they look but it won't happen overnight. Even going to the gym four times a week won't result in a radical transformation if you don't work hard while you're there or aren't eating well.

Q What happens if I miss a session?

A You need to train four times a week and not on more than two consecutive days. This isn't a programme you can dip in and out of – if you do, you'll fail to achieve your objectives. Pick a good time to start when you can dedicate yourself to the whole 12-week challenge.

Q Do I need to stick to the eating plan?

A Yes – any deviation from what is laid out will harm your chances of getting the very best results possible. You need to get it into your head that you're eating for your muscles, not your tastebuds.
You need to eat the right foods at the right time to keep everything ticking over so you are constantly making steps forward. If you don't follow the diet 100%, then don't expect 100% of the results.

Q How long should each workout last?

A Each workout in this programme should last less than an hour. If it's taking any longer than that, you're not sticking to the detailed rest periods. Equally, if you find you're done in less than 45 minutes you're not sticking to the right tempos. Both are just as important to your transformation as sets and reps, so pay close attention to get them right.

Q Can I turn fat into muscle?

A Fat and muscle are two totally different types of tissue, so it's impossible for one to turn into the other. Muscle is active tissue that burns calories, while fat tissues store excess energy.
When you train hard, it's possible to burn away fat and build muscle, giving the appearance that one has turned into the other, but this isn't actually the case.

KNOW YOUR MUSCLES

There are over 600 muscles in the human body. These are the major ones you'll be targeting during your workouts

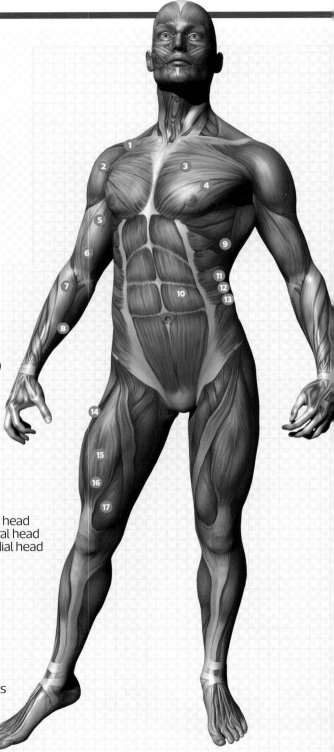

Deltoids
❶ Medial deltoid (middle)
❷ Anterior deltoid (front)

Pectorals
❸ Pectoralis major
❹ Pectoralis minor (beneath the pectoralis major)

Biceps
❺ Biceps brachii
❻ Brachialis
❼ Brachioradialis

Forearms
❽ Flexor carpi radialis

Abdominals
❾ Serratus anterior
❿ Rectus abdominis
⓫ External obliques
⓬ Internal obliques (beneath external obliques)
⓭ Transverse abdominis (beneath internal obliques)

Quadriceps
⓮ Vastus lateralis
⓯ Rectus femoris
⓰ Vastus intermedius (beneath rectus femoris)
⓱ Vastus medialis

Traps
❶ Trapezius

Back
❷ Teres major
❸ Rhomboid (beneath trapezius)

Deltoids
❹ Rotator cuff (beneath deltoids)
❺ Posterior deltoid (back)

Lats
❻ Latissimus dorsi

Triceps
❼ Triceps brachii long head
❽ Triceps brachii lateral head
❾ Triceps brachii medial head

Lower back
❿ Erector spinae

Glutes
⓫ Gluteus maximus

Hamstrings
⓬ Biceps femoris
⓭ Semitendinosus
⓮ Semimembranosus

Calves
⓯ Gastrocnemius
⓰ Soleus

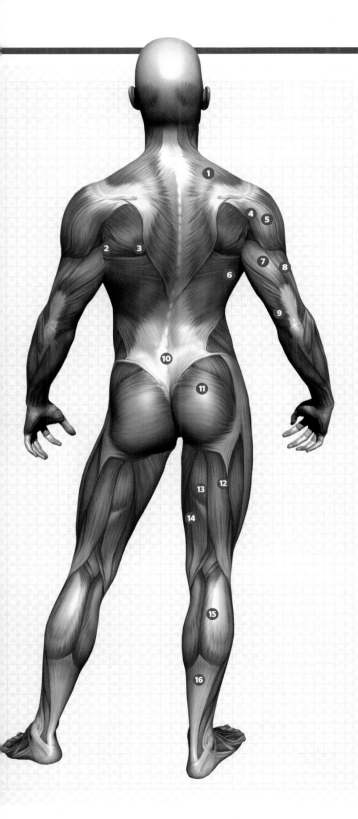

WARMING UP
Get your warm-up right and be stronger

Dashing straight from the changing room into your first set without warming up isn't just dangerous, it's also stupid. A proper warm-up not only prepares your muscles for what lies ahead, helping to prevent injury. It also fires up your central nervous system so your muscles contract quicker, making you stronger, when the session begins.

If you thought the best way to warm up was five minutes on the treadmill, it's time to think again. How can a gentle jog prime your muscles for a hard weights session, especially if you're training your upper body? Here's what you need to do.

The warm-up
The most effective way to warm up your muscles is to perform progressively heavier versions of the moves you'll be doing in the workout itself. Start with a few reps at an easy weight then gradually increase the weight, keeping the reps low to minimise fatigue, until you reach your target workout weight.

Here is a formula you can use to ensure that you select the right weight. It's based on a target workout weight of 100kg for 10 reps.

WARM-UP SET 1
8 reps at 30% (30kg), minimal rest
WARM-UP SET 2
5 reps at 50% (50kg), 30-60sec rest
WARM-UP SET 3
3 reps at 70% (70kg), 45-75sec rest
WARM-UP SET 4
2 reps at 85% (85kg), 60-75sec rest
WARM-UP SET 5
1 rep at 95% (95kg), 60-75sec rest
START FIRST WORK-SET

You only need to do this for the first two moves. For all subsequent moves for the same or a similar body part, select a weight about two-thirds of your target and perform four to six reps to get the motor pattern right.

If you're moving to a new muscle group, do this warm-up sequence again. If chin-ups, pull-ups or dips are in the first two moves, use a resistance machine to warm up.

The cool-down
Cooling down is simple for this programme: drink a protein shake and hit the shower. That's all.

ACTIVATION ADVANTAGE
Explosive movements before your initial workouts can further activate your central nervous system to elicit greater reaction and force from your muscles. Before pushing exercises, hurl a medicine ball at the ground as hard as possible, do a couple of clap press-ups or unleash a couple of left and right hooks at a punch bag. Before lower-body exercises, a couple of hard kicks to a heavy bag will do the trick or complete a few jump squats.

HOW MUSCLES GROW

The simple science behind adding muscle mass and making your body bigger and stronger

Muscle growth is essentially your body responding to the stress of weight training. It's thinking, 'That was hard. I'd better do something about that so it's not as difficult next time.'

When you perform weight-training exercises, you create microscopic tears in your muscles. Your body's response to this 'microtrauma' of the muscle cells is to overcompensate by not just repairing the damaged tissue but by adding more.

In this way your muscles become bigger and stronger and so the risk of future damage is minimised. It also means you should progressively increase the weight you lift, because your muscles quickly adapt to deal with the original stress to which they've been exposed.

It's also thought that this damage to your muscle fibres is the reason for the soreness and stiffness you feel in your muscles in the days after a tough workout, which is known as delayed onset muscle soreness or DOMS. And it's why you should always leave at least 48 hours between workout sessions that target the same muscle group. If you train again before your muscles have been repaired and rebuilt, you won't be as strong and you run the risk of injuring yourself.

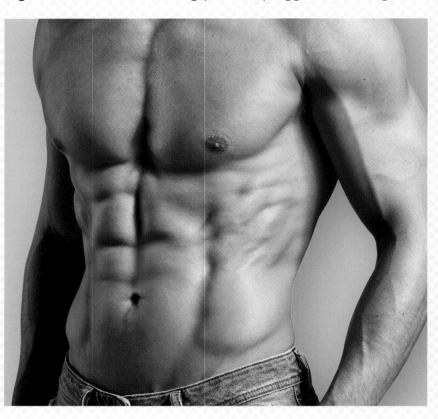

ANATOMY OF A MUSCLE
What your muscles are made of

Muscles are constructed of bundles of fibres contained within protective sheaths called fascia, which are then themselves bundled together. The biggest bundle is the muscle itself. Next in line are the fascicles, which contain the long, single-celled muscle fibres. Muscle fibres are then sub-divided into myofibrils, which are divided again into bundles of myofilaments, made up from chains of sarcomeres.

❶ TENDON
Strong tissue that connects muscle to bone.

❷ EPIMYSIUM
A layer of connective tissue that encases the entire muscle.

❸ ENDOMYSIUM
Connective tissue that covers the muscle fibres and also contains capillaries and nerves.

❹ PERIMYSIUM
A layer of connective tissue that

bundles together between ten and several hundred individual muscle fibres into fascicles.

❺ FASCICLE
A bundle of individual muscle fibres.

❻ MYOFILAMENTS
The smallest fibre bundles in your muscles.

❼ MUSCLE FIBRE
There are two main types of muscle fibre: type 1 or slow-

How muscles work

What happens during a workout and while you rest? Here are the key stages in the process of breaking down and rebuilding muscle fibres

1 THE WARM-UP

An increased heart rate pumps blood to your muscles, warming them up and allowing them to extend fully. It also supplies the muscle fibres with oxygen.

2 LOADING THE MUSCLE

At the start of each rep, your muscles are under load and stretched. As a result, your heart pumps more blood into the protective sheaths that surround the muscle fibres, supplying oxygen and nutrients to these fibres.

3 SPARKING YOUR NERVOUS SYSTEM

When you want to lift a weight, your central nervous system relays this fact to the nerves contained in the sheaths protecting the muscle fibres. In turn, they tell the muscle fibres to contract and lift the weight. If you're doing the exercise correctly, your muscles will activate in a particular sequence and your central nervous system adapts to this. As you repeat the workout over time, your nerves get more efficient so you can do more reps or lift more weight.

4 CHEMICAL REACTIONS

Adenosine triphosphate (ATP) is the immediate energy source for muscle contraction. It's broken down within the body's cells to release energy. The cells' creatine, phosphate and glycogen reserves are also converted into ATP. This process creates lactic acid as a by-product.

5 FEELING THE BURN

Once the glycogen stores in the cells have been depleted and lactic acid has built up, the muscle can't work efficiently, so you need to rest. While you rest, aerobic (oxygen-based) muscle respiration occurs, converting lactic acid back into glycogen to give you energy for the next set.

6 SUCCESSFUL FAILURE

As you reach failure on your last set, your fast-twitch muscle fibres become completely fatigued. Microscopic tears (or 'microtears') are created in the myofilaments, the smallest fibre bundles in your muscles.

7 REPAIR AND GROWTH

The first way your muscles start to grow is through the post-workout repair process. Your body repairs the microtears by adding the amino acids actin and myosin to the myofilaments, which also causes them to grow in size.

Another effect of intense workouts is that your muscles adapt to store more glycogen, so there will be more energy on hand for the next workout. This also has the happy side effect of making the muscles increase in size slightly.

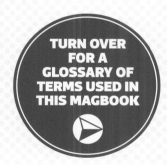

TURN OVER FOR A GLOSSARY OF TERMS USED IN THIS MAGBOOK

twitch, which are slow to fatigue and best suited to endurance; and type 2 or fast-twitch, which fatigue quickly and are suited to fast, explosive movements.

❽ BLOOD VESSEL

Blood vessels come in three types: arteries, which transport oxygenated blood away from the heart; veins, which transport deoxygenated blood back to the heart; and capillaries, which enable the exchange of nutrients and waste products between the blood and tissues.

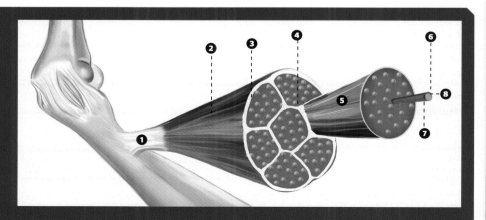

GLOSSARY

Simple explanations of these common workout terms

Compound lift

A compound lift is an exercise where there is movement in two or more different joints. Good examples are the squat (movement at the hip and knee joints) and shoulder press (movement at the shoulder and elbow joints).

Such lifts should form the basis of all programmes where increasing muscle size and strength is the objective because they recruit more of the muscle fibres responsible for the development of size and strength.

Concentric contractions

During concentric contractions the muscle shortens while generating force. In general, concentric muscle actions are responsible for the 'raising' part of an exercise, such as the biceps shortening as you lift a dumbbell from your side to shoulder height during a biceps curl.

Drop set

A series of sets of the same exercise in which you start with a heavy weight, lift until you reach failure, then drop the weight and go again. Drop sets are typically three such sets performed without rest.

Eccentric contractions

During eccentric contractions the muscle lengthens under tension when controlling a weight. This usually means the 'lowering' part of an exercise, such as the biceps

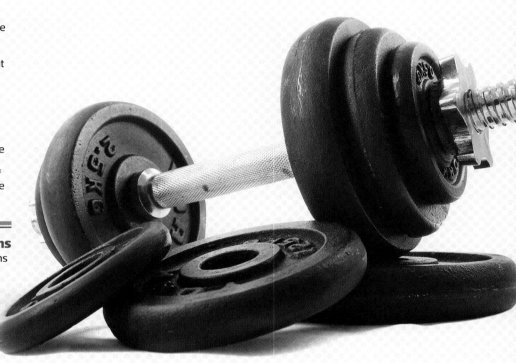

elongating as your control the weight back down to the start position during a biceps curl.

Your muscles are 10–20% stronger during eccentric contractions than concentric contractions, and it is heavy eccentric loads that cause the maximum amount of damage to muscles. That's why it's important to lower a weight slowly and under control: not only does this minimise the risk of injury, it also makes each rep more effective.

Failure

Training to momentary muscular failure is a strategy in which you're unable to lift the weight with correct form on the final rep of your set. This form of overload training shocks your muscles into growing back bigger and stronger, but it's vital you have a spotter on hand when training to failure on big compound lifts to minimise the risk of injury.

Fascia

Fascia, Latin for 'band', is a layer of fibrous connective tissue that surrounds muscles, blood vessels and nerves. It is multilayered, so think of it as a sheath that encases not

only each muscle cell but also each body part and even your entire body. If your fascia is too tight, your body will have a harder time stretching it to create the room necessary for a muscle to grow bigger.

Glycogen

A type of energy stored in the muscles and liver, glycogen is the primary fuel used by your body in this programme. Too little glycogen and you can start to both look and feel 'flat'.

Hypertrophy

The Greek word for 'excess

nourishment', hypertrophy is an increase in the volume of a muscle (or organ) owing to the enlargement of its component cells. Hypertrophy occurs through either sarcoplasmic or myofibrillar growth (see below), or a combination.

Isolation lift
An isolation move is where there is movement at one joint only. Examples include a biceps curl (movement at the elbow joint only) and leg extension (movement at the knee joint only). These exercises are great for the end of your workouts when you can really work a target muscle group to fatigue.

Isometric contractions
During isometric contractions, a muscle generates force without changing length. Typical examples include your entire abdominal region during a plank, or the muscles of the hand and wrist when you grip an object.

Such contractions aren't as effective for building and maintaining muscle mass when compared with concentric and eccentric contractions, but they should still form an important element of your training programme, especially for core work.

Muscle pump
The pump occurs when your muscles become engorged with blood after you have repeatedly shortened and lengthened a muscle. Typically this occurs when using weight training but sometimes it can be achieved simply by flexing your muscles repeatedly as hard as possible.

Myofibrillar growth
This is when a muscle gets bigger because of an increase in the number and size of cells within that muscle.

Peak contraction
A peak contraction occurs when the muscle has a full contraction against resistance for the entire range of motion, as opposed to where it might get 'easier' as the rep is completed. Contrast a peak contraction exercise such as a cable preacher curl with a barbell squat, for example.

Reps
An abbreviation of repetition, one rep is the completion of a given exercise from start to finish through a full range of motion. The number of reps per set can vary from one to more than 20, depending on your training goals.

Rest interval
Taking rest between sets and exercises allows your muscles to replenish their energy stores. In this programme, rest intervals are manipulated in different ways to help provide ongoing muscular stimulus.

Sarcoplasmic growth
This is when muscle size increases because of an increase in the volume of sarcoplasmic fluid within the muscle cells.

Sets
A set is a given number of reps (see above) performed consecutively without rest. The number of sets performed of each exercise can vary depending on the workout and its specific goals, but three or four sets is considered most effective if you want to build muscle mass.

Supercompensation
This is the period after training and recovery during which you are fitter and stronger than before training. Training again in this supercompensation window will result in further gains in strength, size and fitness.

Equally, training before this window can result in overtraining, where you actually become weaker, while training once it has closed results in the loss of your ability to make additional gains.

Superset
A superset is two or more moves done back to back with little or no rest between exercises. They are a great way to shake up your existing training regime as they shock your muscles into growing because of the increased workload and they allow you to train with more volume in a shorter period of time, improving your muscles' ability to work harder with less rest. Supersets in this programme are detailed by naming exercises 1a and 1b or 2a and 2b and so on, depending on where they appear in the workout order. Supersets can contain up to six moves and be labelled up to the letter 'f'.

Tempo
This is the speed at which you lift and lower a weight during a rep. The slower the tempo, the longer your muscles are exposed to the stress of managing the weight. This is called 'time under tension'.

Tempo is detailed by a four-digit code, such as 4010. The first number is the time in seconds the weight is lowered; the second is the time in seconds the move is held at the bottom position; the third is the time in seconds that the weight it lifted (if 'X' is shown this means lift explosively); and the final digit is the time in seconds the weight is held at the top of the move.

Time under tension
Time under tension is the duration in seconds your muscles are controlling a weight through a range of motion, as in a squat or bench press. It's dictated by the tempo of each rep and how many reps in a given set, with the total time the sum of all the reps and the eccentric and concentric movements plus the time at the top and bottom of each rep.

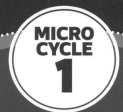

MICRO CYCLE 1

WORKOUTS
1 TO 8

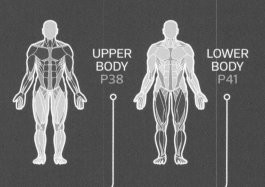

UPPER BODY
P38

LOWER BODY
P41

| 1 | 3 | 5 | 7 | 2 | 4 | 6 | 8 |

STRONG START

Ignite your muscle-building mission with these workouts

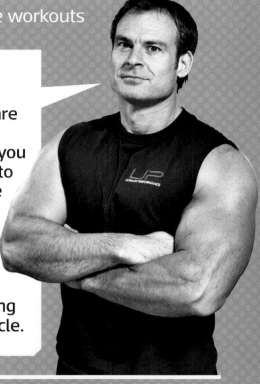

This first eight-workout microcycle is an 'intensification' phase to get you as strong as possible as quickly as possible. The workouts are built around low reps with heavy weights.

By beginning with strength-based workouts you are training your muscles and nervous system to cope with stress. This will enable you to handle more weight for more reps in the next microcycle, where the focus shifts towards pure hypertrophy, or muscle building.

There are two workouts here: an upper-body session and a lower-body session. This is a tough start, but nail it and you'll have a strong foundation from which to start packing on muscle.

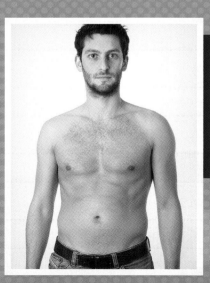

MICROCYCLE 1

WEIGHT
72.3kg

BODY FAT PERCENTAGE
16.5%

HOW TO DO THESE WORKOUTS

You'll perform four sessions a week for two weeks. Do workout 1 (upper body) and 2 (lower body) in order, then repeat this sequence for workouts 3 to 8 before advancing to the next microcycle. Increase the weight for each session without losing form. Don't work out on more than two consecutive days.

Upper body

EXERCISE	SETS	REPS	TEMPO	REST
SET 1				
1a Chin-up	4	8	4010	90sec
1b Incline bench press	4	8	4010	90sec
SET 2				
2a Rack deadlift	4	8	2111	90sec
2b Triceps dip	4	8	4010	90sec
SET 3				
3a High pull	4	8	2110	45sec
3b Decline plank with alternate foot touch	4	25	2010	45sec

1a Chin-up

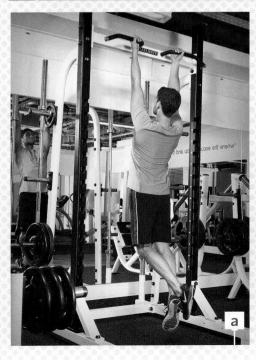
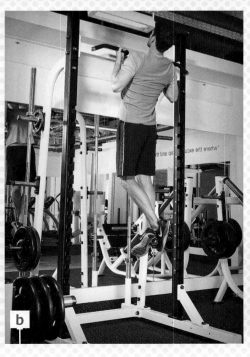

a

b

- Grab the bar with an underhand grip with your hands close together.
- Start from a dead hang with your arms fully extended.
- Pull yourself up by squeezing your lats together.
- Once your chin is higher than your hands, lower yourself back to the start.

TRAINER TIP

- Don't think chin-up, think chest-up: squeeze your lats and biceps so that your chest hits the bar, and don't reach forward with your chin.

1b Incline bench press

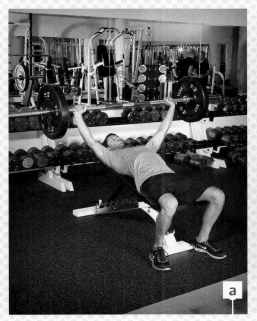
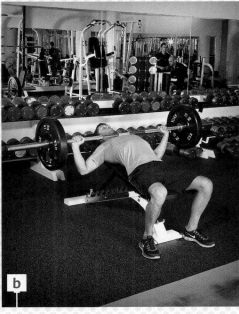

a   b

○ Lie on a bench set at a 30–45° angle holding a barbell with an overhand grip.

○ Keep your feet flat on the floor and your back against the bench.

○ Slowly lower the weight down to your chest, flaring your elbows out to the sides, until the bar touches your chest.

○ Press the weight directly above your head but don't lock out your elbows.

TRAINER TIP

○ Don't try to press the bar with your shoulders. Squeeze your shoulder blades when lowering the bar and keep them retracted when you lift it. You'll be more stable and therefore stronger.

2a Rack deadlift

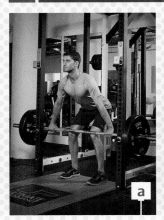
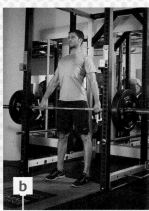

a   b

○ Set the safety bars on a squat rack to mid-knee level.

○ With the barbell resting on the bars, take a wide grip with your core braced, your back flat and your shoulders retracted and over the bar.

○ Use your glutes to power the initial lift, pushing down through your heels.

○ Keep the bar close to your body and, as it passes your knees, push your hips forward. Then lower the weight back down so it just touches the bars and repeat.

2b Triceps dip

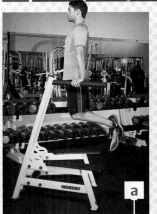
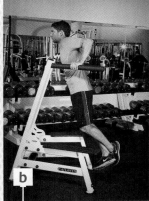

a   b

○ Grip parallel bars, keeping your body upright.

○ With your elbows pointing straight back, lower your body as far down as you can comfortably go without stressing your shoulders.

○ Keep your core braced and don't swing your legs for momentum.

○ Press back up powerfully but don't lock out your elbows at the top.

3a High pull

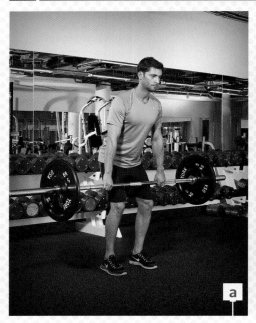
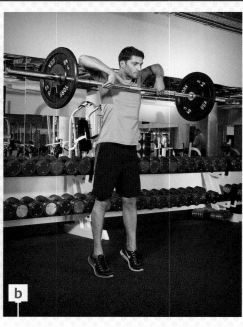

a   b

- Stand tall holding a barbell at hip height with an overhand grip slightly narrower than shoulder-width.
- Shrug the bar up towards your chin, leading with your elbows, which are pointing to the ceiling.
- Slowly lower the bar back to the start.

TRAINER TIP

- The trick with this complicated exercise is to concentrate on throwing your hips forward as you lift the bar. If you master this then everything else will click into place.

3b Decline plank with alternate foot touch

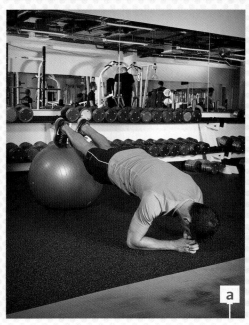
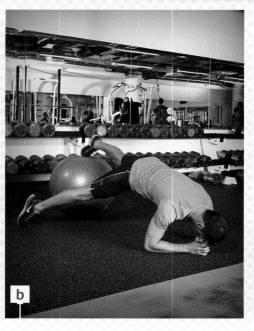

a   b

- With your feet on a raised platform, bench or gym ball, hold your body in a straight line from head to heels with your elbows beneath your shoulders and your head looking down.
- Hold the position and, without letting your hips sag, lift one foot up and out to the side, then lower it to the floor.
- Once you've touched the ground, return that leg to the start position and repeat with your other leg.

TRAINER TIP

- Keep your core braced throughout every rep for the entire set to keep your abs under tension for as long as possible.

Lower body

EXERCISE	SETS	REPS	TEMPO	REST
SET 1				
1a Squat	4*	8	4010	90sec
1b Lying hamstring curl	6**	6	4010	90sec
SET 2				
2a Incline back extension	4	8	4011	0sec
2b Calf raise	4	12	4010	90sec
SET 3				
3a Hanging leg raise	4	15	3010	0sec
3b Decline dumbbell crunch	4	12	3010	90sec

* Perform a four-rep max set for the last set, then reduce the weight and perform six reps, then reduce it again for another six reps, so that the total number of reps in this final set is 16.

** You will perform two more sets of lying hamstring curls than squats in this superset. Take 90sec rest between these two additional sets.

1a Squat

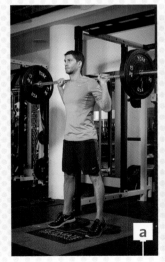
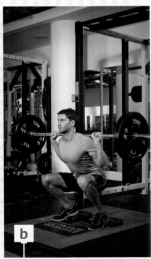

- Rest the bar against the back of your shoulders – not on your neck – and hold it with an overhand grip slightly wider than your shoulders. Keep your elbows pointing down.
- Your feet should be just wider than shoulder-width apart

and your toes pointing outwards slightly.
- Squat down until your thighs are at least parallel to the floor. The deeper you can squat, the better.
- Drive back up through your heels.

1b Lying hamstring curl

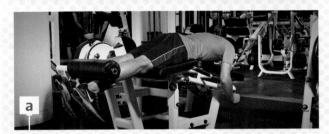
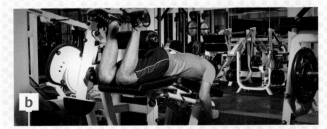

- Lie on the machine, following its instructions to position yourself correctly and safely.
- With the pad against the back of your lower calves, raise it by contracting your hamstrings.
- Return slowly to the start.

TRAINER TIP

- Don't swing the weight up and down. Squeeze it up and slowly lower it. Don't be afraid to reduce the weight – tempo is the key here.

2a Incline back extension

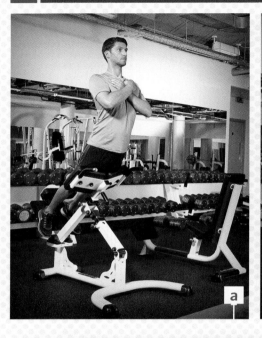
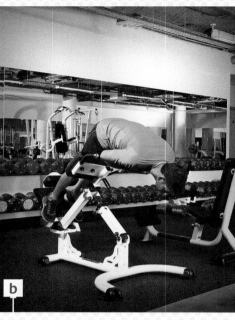

- Position yourself on the bench with your feet and thighs supported.
- With your hands touching your temples or crossed across your chest and your core braced, lower your torso as far as is comfortable.
- Use your lower back muscles to return you to the start position.

2b Calf raise

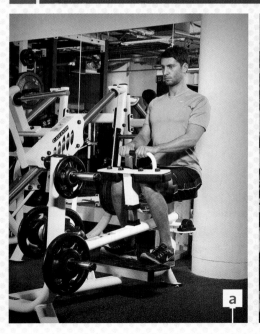
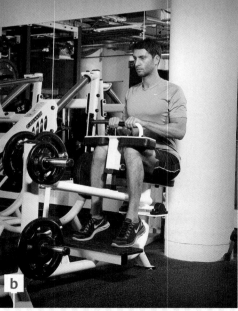

- Sit on the machine – having adjusted the weight plates or stack, depending on the equipment – with your toes on the platform.
- Release the safety catch and go up on to your tiptoes, keeping your body stable.
- Pause briefly before returning to the start, ensuring that your heel goes below the level of the platform for a full range of motion.

TRAINER TIP

- You need to get a really good stretch in your calf muscles to make them work hard and force them to grow.

3a Hanging leg raise

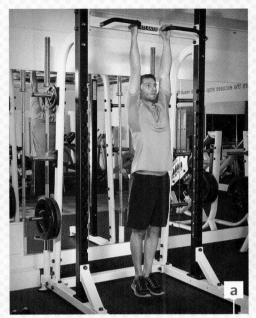
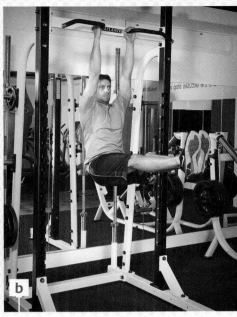

a b

- Hang from a bar with your body straight.
- Keeping your legs straight, use your lower abs to raise them up until they're parallel with the ground.
- Lower back down to the start position.

TRAINER TIP

- Don't just swing your legs up and down: it uses momentum and not your muscles so it's a complete waste of time.

3b Decline dumbbell crunch

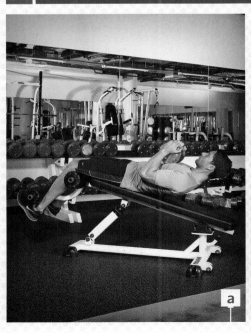
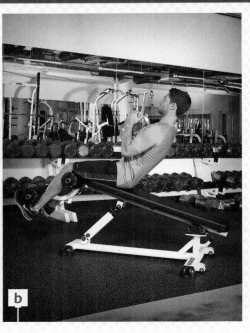

a b

- Lie on a decline bench holding a dumbbell on your chest.
- Contract your abs to lift your shoulders up and curl your chest towards your knees.
- Pause at the top of the move, squeeze your abs and lower slowly to the start.

WORKOUTS 9 TO 17

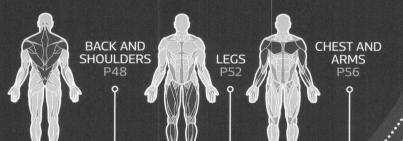

BACK AND SHOULDERS
P48

LEGS
P52

CHEST AND ARMS
P56

| 9 | 12 | 15 | | 10 | 13 | 16 | | 11 | 14 | 17 |

MUSCLE UP

These workouts will pack on muscle size while burning fat

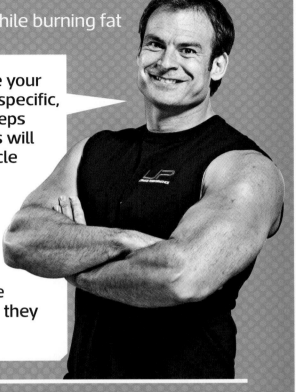

After the initial strength-building microcycle your muscles are ready for a more hypertrophy-specific, or muscle-building, phase. The number of reps you perform will increase while rest periods will decrease, so the volume of work each muscle group must handle increases significantly.

This phase also moves to a three-way split: back and shoulders; legs; and chest and arms, and includes drops sets. The extra volume increases blood flow to the target muscles, ups the rate at which your body burns calories and allows you to cause maximum damage to your muscle fibres so they grow back bigger and stronger.

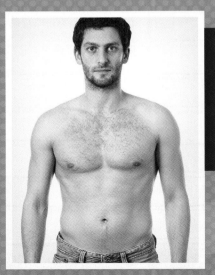

MICROCYCLE 2

WEIGHT
72.8kg

BODY FAT
PERCENTAGE
13.3%

HOW TO DO THESE WORKOUTS

You'll perform four sessions a week for two weeks. Do workout 9 (back and shoulders), 10 (legs) and 11 (chest and arms) in order, before repeating this sequence with workouts 12 through to 17 then advancing to the next microcycle. Increase the weight for each session without losing form. Never work out on more than two consecutive days.

Back and shoulders

EXERCISE	SETS	REPS	TEMPO	REST
SET 1				
1a **Pull-up**	3	12	3111	60sec
1b **Seated barbell shoulder press**	3	12	4010	60sec
SET 2				
2a **Band pull**	3	15	20X1	10sec
2b **Bent-over row**	3	12	3010	75sec
SET 3				
3a **Dumbbell pull-over**	3	10	4111	0sec
3b **Close-grip lat pull-down**	3	10	3011	10sec
3c **Face pull**	3	15	2010	90sec
SET 4				
4a **Lateral raise**	3	15	2010	45sec
4b **Incline bench shrug**	3	15	2011	45sec

1a Pull-up

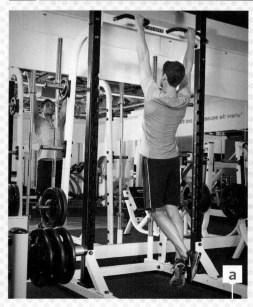
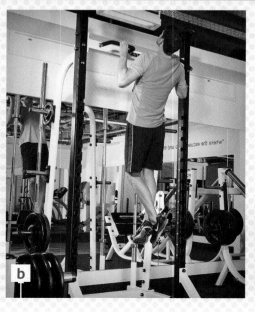

- Grab the bar with an overhand grip with your hands shoulder-width apart.
- Start from a dead hang with your arms fully extended.
- Pull yourself up by squeezing your lats together.
- Once your chin is higher than your hands pause briefly, then slowly lower yourself back to the start.

TRAINER TIP

- Your arms shouldn't be directly pulling you up. Drive the elbows back and squeeze your upper back muscles.

1b Seated barbell shoulder press

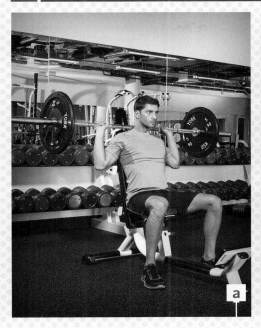

a

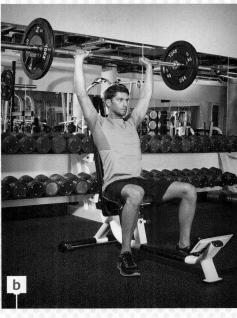

b

- Sit on an upright bench with a barbell on your upper chest, gripping it with hands shoulder-width apart.
- Keep your chest upright and your core muscles braced.
- Press the bar directly upwards until your arms are extended overhead.
- Lower the bar back down behind your neck then press back up.

TRAINER TIP

- To improve stability, squeeze your shoulder blades during the lowering phase then press back up powerfully from the bottom of the move.

2a Band pull

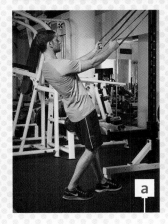

a

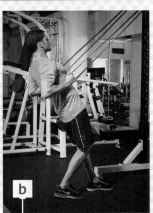

b

- Attach two resistance bands to the top of a squat rack or pull-up bar and hold the ends, one in each hand.
- Leaning back slightly, pull the bands down explosively, leading with your elbows, until your hands are just below chest height.
- Return slowly to the start position.

2b Bent-over row

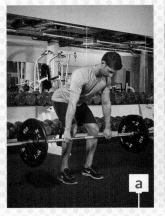

a

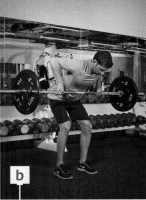

b

- Start with your core braced, your back straight and your shoulder blades retracted.
- Bend your knees slightly and lean forward from the hips.
- Grip the bar with your hands just wider than shoulder-width apart letting them hang at knee level.
- Pull the bar up to your lower sternum, retracting your shoulder blades to allow the bar to come up to your chest, then lower the bar slowly back to the start.

3a Dumbbell pull-over

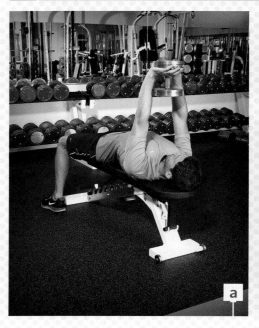
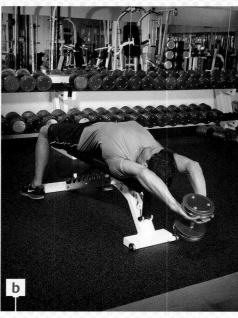

- Lie flat on a bench with your head and shoulders supported and your feet flat on the floor.
- Hold a single dumbbell over your chest with both hands and engage your core.
- Slowly lower the weight behind your head, keeping a slight bend in your elbows. Don't arch your back.
- Raise the weight back over your head to the start position.

3b Close-grip lat pull-down

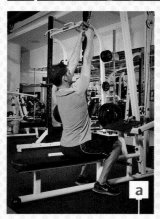
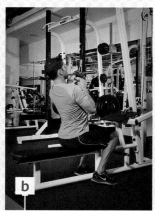

- Sit on the seat and hold a D-handle attachment with both hands.
- Look forward, retract your shoulder blades and keep your torso upright.
- Pull the bar down in front of you until it reaches your upper chest. Don't lean back to aid the movement.
- Squeeze your lats at the bottom of the move and return the bar slowly to the top.

3c Face pull

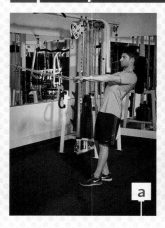
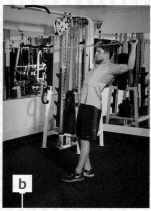

- Hold a double-rope attachment that's connected to the high pulley on a cable machine.
- Start with arms fully extended with palms facing the floor.
- Pull the handles towards your head – keeping your upper arms parallel to the floor – so that the handles go to either side of your face.
- Return to the start.

4a Lateral raise

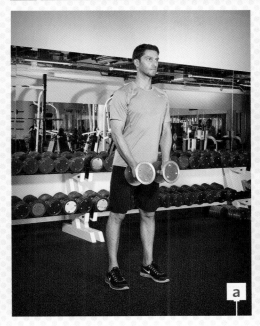
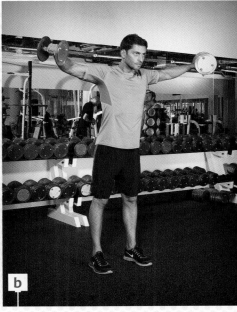

a   b

- Stand tall with your core braced and your feet apart, holding a light dumbbell in each hand by your sides with your palms facing one another.
- Keeping a slight bend in your elbows, raise the weights out to the sides using your muscles and not momentum.
- Stop at shoulder height, pause for a second, then slowly return to the start.

TRAINER TIP

- Rotate your whole arm, not just your hands, during this move – it's this action that affects deltoid activation.

4b Incline bench shrug

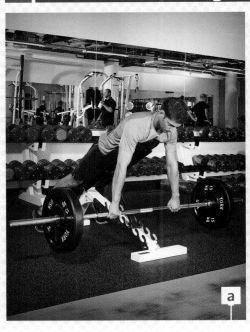
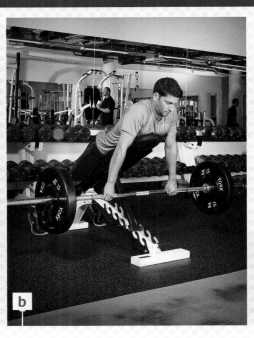

a   b

- Lie chest-first on an incline bench holding a barbell with a wide, overhand grip.
- Keeping your chest on the bench, shrug the barbell up using your upper back muscles.
- Return to the start.

TRAINER TIP

- Don't let your arms get in on the act during this move. Concentrate on pulling with your upper back.

Legs

EXERCISE	SETS	REPS	TEMPO	REST
SET 1				
1a Safety bar squat+	2	4	6010	90sec
1b Kneeling hamstring curl	4*	4	4010	90sec
SET 2				
2 Safety bar squat+	2	20	3011	180sec
SET 3				
3a Incline back extension	3	12	3012	10sec
3b Reverse hyperextension	3	10	3011	10sec
SET 4				
4a Dumbbell step-up	3	15	2010	180sec
4b Leg press	3	45**	2010	60sec
SET 5				
5 Farmer's walk	3	40m	X	90sec

+
If your gym doesn't have a safety squat bar perform back squats instead.

*
You'll perform two more sets of lying hamstring curls than safety bar squats in this superset. Rest for 90sec between these extra sets.

* *
Perform 15 reps with your feet 12cm apart, 15 with feet hip-width apart, then 15 reps with feet 10cm wider than hip-width for a total of 45 per set.

1a Safety bar squat

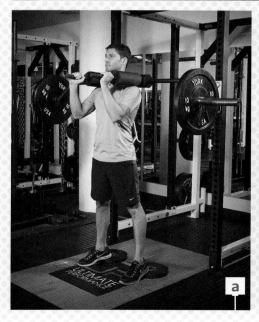
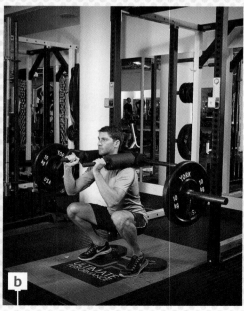

a

b

- Rest the bar against the back of your shoulders – not on your neck – and hold the handles, keeping your elbows up so your upper arms are parallel to the floor.
- Your feet should be just wider than shoulder-width apart with your toes pointing outwards slightly.
- Squat down until your thighs are at least parallel to the floor. The deeper you can squat, the better.
- Drive back up through your heels.

TRAINER TIP

- If you have poor flexibility then elevate your heels on weight plates to allow a deeper range of motion.

1b Kneeling hamstring curl

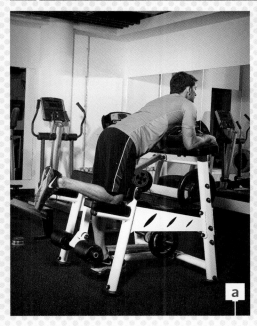
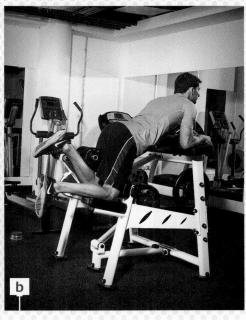

a   b

- Kneel over the machine, following its instructions to position yourself correctly and safely.
- With the pad against the back of your lower calf, raise it up by contracting your hamstrings.
- Return slowly to the start.
- Complete all reps then switch legs.

2 Safety bar squat

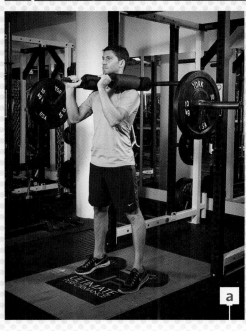
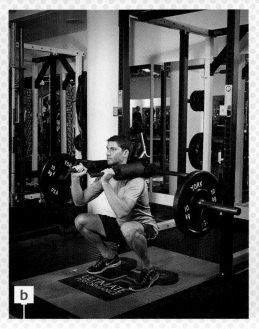

a   b

- Rest the bar against the back of your shoulders – not on your neck – and hold the handles, keeping your elbows up so your upper arms are parallel to the floor.
- Your feet should be just wider than shoulder-width apart with your toes pointing outwards slightly.
- Squat down until your thighs are at least parallel to the floor. The deeper you can squat, the better.
- Drive back up through your heels.

TRAINER TIP

- Yes, more squats. This isn't a mistake: these two hard extra sets will really test your legs, glutes and core.

3a Incline back extension

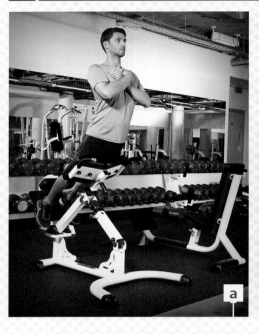
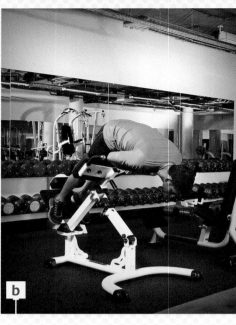

- Position yourself on the bench with your feet and thighs supported.
- With your hands touching your temples and you core braced, lower your torso as far as is comfortable.
- Use your lower back muscles to return you to the start.

3b Reverse hyperextension

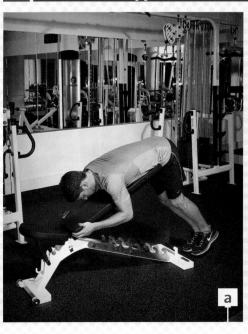
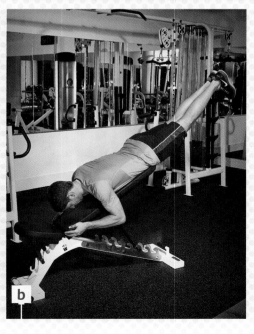

- Lie face down on an incline bench with your chest supported so that your body forms a V-shape with the bend at your hips.
- Raise your legs straight up so that your body forms a straight line from head to heels.
- Lower your legs back down to the start, but don't let them touch the floor.

4a Dumbbell step-up

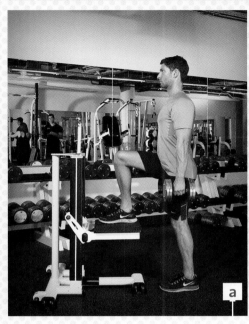

a

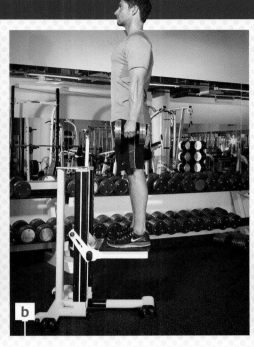

b

- O Stand in front of a platform set at knee height holding a dumbbell in each hand.
- O Keep one foot on the platform and step up and back down with the other.
- O Switch legs and repeat.

TRAINER TIP

- O Bang the sole of your working foot on the platform for greater activation of your hamstrings and glutes.

4b Leg press

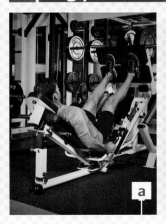

a

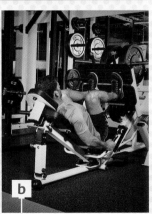

b

- O Sit on the machine, following its instructions to position yourself correctly and safely.
- O Release the lock then slowly lower the platform towards you by bending your knees.
- O Pause briefly at the bottom then push through your heels

to straighten your legs and return to the start.

5 Farmer's walk

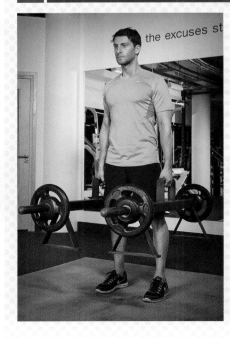

- O Stand in front of a long, clear pathway, holding a weighted bar or dumbbell in each hand.
- O Keeping your core braced, walk as quickly as you can down the track.
- O At the end, turn around and walk back quickly to the start.

Chest and arms

EXERCISE	SETS	REPS	TEMPO	REST
SET 1				
1 Incline dumbbell bench press	3	12*	4010	90sec
SET 2				
2 Guillotine press	3	10*	4010	90sec
SET 3				
3a Decline bench press+	3	12	3010	60sec
3b EZ-bar preacher curl	3	12	4010	60sec
SET 4				
4a Incline hammer curl	3	10	3010	45sec
4b Decline EZ-bar triceps press	3	12	3110	45sec
SET 5				
5a Cable triceps press-down	2	30**	2010	0sec
5b Close-grip cable biceps curl	2	24**	2010	0sec

+
If your gym has chains, attach them at each end of the barbell to work your muscles harder.

✳
The last set is a drop set. Perform the reps, then reduce the weight by 15% and do them again. Repeat the process once more, and rest.

✳✳
Every set is a three-part drop set. Do a third of the reps, then reduce the weight by 15% for the next third and reduce by 15% again for the final third.

1 | Incline dumbbell bench press

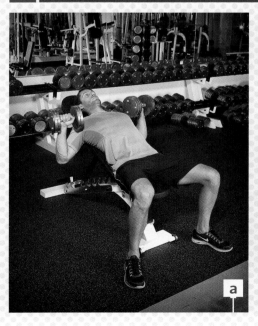
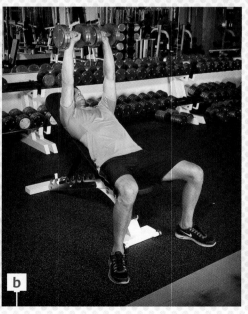

- Lie on a bench set at a 45° angle holding a dumbbell in each hand at shoulder-height.
- Keep your feet flat on the floor and your back against the bench.
- Press the weight directly above your head but don't lock out your elbows at the top.
- Slowly lower the weight back down to your chest, flaring your elbows out to the side.

TRAINER TIP

- If you have shoulder trouble, turn your palms to face each other and tuck your elbows in at the bottom of the move.

2 | Guillotine press

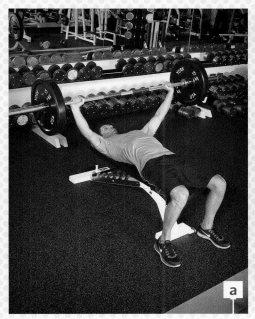

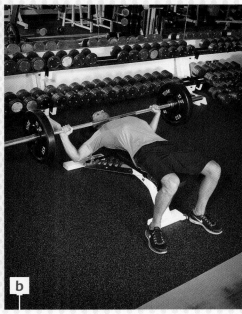

a

b

- Lie on the bench with your feet on the floor, directly under your knees.
- Your head, upper back and glutes should be flat against the bench.
- Hold the bar with an overhand grip shoulder-width apart.
- Slowly lower the bar to your neck, taking your elbows out to 90°, until the bar almost touches you.
- Drive your feet hard into the floor and push the bar back strongly to the start position.

TRAINER TIP

- Focus on stretching and squeezing your chest muscles (as you lower and raise the weight) as much as possible.

3a | Decline bench press

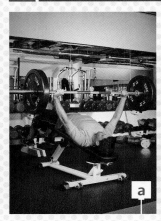

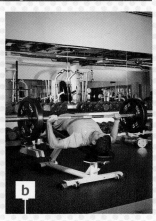

a

b

- Lie on a decline bench with your feet on the floor, directly under your knees.
- Your head, upper back and glutes should be flat against the bench.
- Hold the bar with an overhand grip shoulder-width apart.
- Slowly lower the bar, taking your elbows out to 90°, until the bar is almost touching the middle of your chest.
- Drive your feet hard into the floor and push the bar back strongly to the start position.

3b | EZ-bar preacher curl

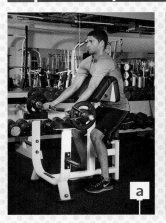

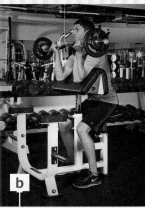

a

b

- Sit at a preacher bench holding an EZ-bar with an underhand grip.
- Keeping your elbows on the bench, curl the bar up towards your chin.
- Slowly lower the bar back to the start.
- Avoid rocking back and forth to generate momentum, which takes the emphasis away from the biceps.

4a Incline hammer curl

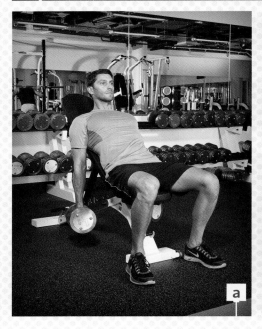
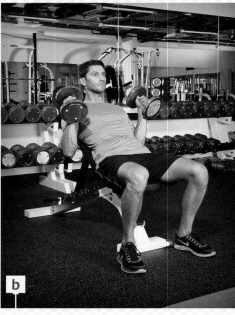

- Sit on an incline bench holding a dumbbell in each hand with your palms facing each other.
- Keeping your elbows close to your side, slowly raise both dumbbells up to shoulder height, squeezing your biceps at the top of the move.
- Slowly return the weight to the start position.

TRAINER TIP

- Try to stretch out your triceps as hard as you can at the bottom of the move, and squeeze your biceps hard at the top.

4b Decline EZ-bar triceps press

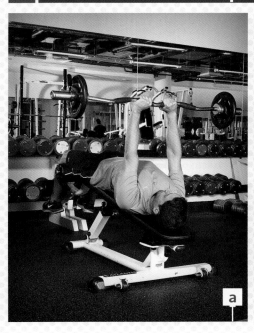
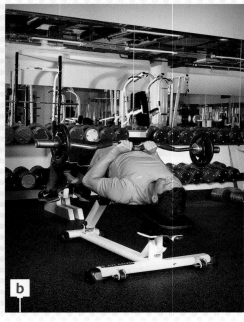

- Lie flat on a decline bench holding an EZ-bar with a close, overhand grip. Aim to have a fist-sized gap between your hands.
- Keep your head, shoulders and back supported by the bench with your core braced and feet flat on the floor.
- Lower the bar slowly to your chest, keeping your elbows close to your sides to keep the emphasis on your triceps.
- Push back up powerfully, but don't lock out your elbows.

5a Cable triceps press-down

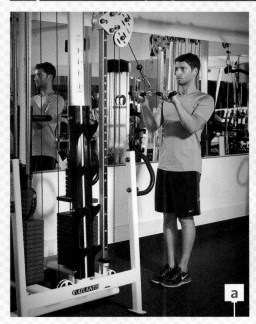

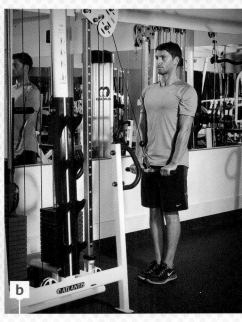

- Stand tall, holding an EZ-bar cable handle attached to the high pulley of a cable machine.
- Keeping your elbows next to your body, press your hands down to straighten your arms.
- Squeeze your triceps at the bottom of the move, then return to the start, squeezing your biceps at the very top.

5b Cable EZ-bar biceps curl

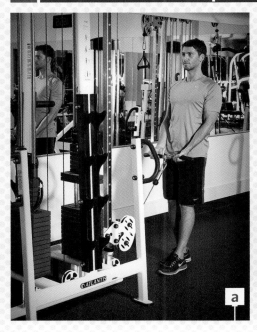

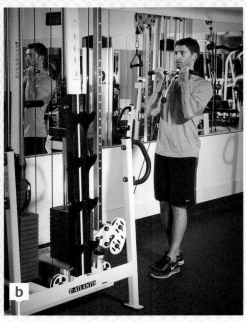

- Stand tall, holding an EZ-bar cable handle attached to the low pulley of a cable machine.
- Keeping your elbows next to your body, curl your hands up to raise the handles towards your chin.
- Squeeze your biceps at the top of the move, then return to the start, squeezing your triceps at the very bottom.

MICRO CYCLE 3

WORKOUTS 18 TO 20

BACK AND
SHOULDERS
P60

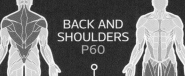

LEGS
P63

CHEST AND
ARMS
P66

18 19 20

SHOCK AND AWE

This short phase destroys your muscles for bigger gains

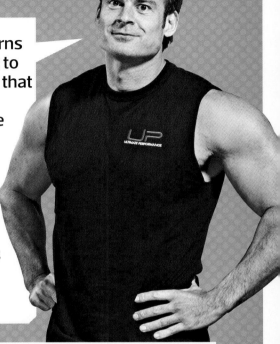

This short microcycle – just three workouts – turns everything on its head. It's a quick, intense blast to give you a break from high-volume sessions so that you bounce back bigger and stronger.

The aim is to cause the most damage possible in the shortest time. There are fewer sets, but more drop sets, forced reps and increased 'intensity'. This gives you a deload, because your joints and nervous system won't be taxed as much as in the previous two microcycles, while still stimulating growth.

Forced reps, drop sets and the other variables are unpleasant but you must attack them with 100% determination and aggression.

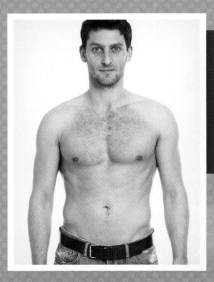

MICROCYCLE 3

WEIGHT
73.5kg

BODY FAT PERCENTAGE
12.8%

HOW TO DO THESE WORKOUTS

Do workout 18 (back and shoulders), 19 (legs) and 20 (chest and arms) in order, before advancing to the next microcycle. Never work out on more than two consecutive days.

Back and shoulders

EXERCISE	SETS	REPS	TEMPO	REST
SET 1				
1 Underhand lat pull-down	2	10	4010	60sec
SET 2				
2 Seated cable row	2	10*	3010	60sec
SET 3				
3 Reverse bench row	1	10*	3010	90sec
SET 4				
4 Seated dumbbell shoulder press	1	15	3010	90sec
SET 5				
5 Cable lateral raise	2	12*	3010	60sec
SET 6				
6 Face pull	2	12*	3010	60sec

* The final set is a drop set. Perform the stated number of reps, then reduce the weight by 15% and do the same number of reps. Repeat this process once more, then rest.

1 | Underhand lat pull-down

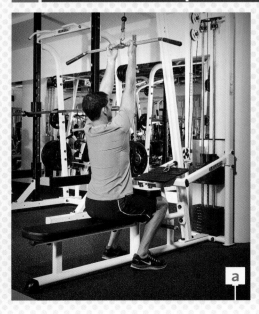
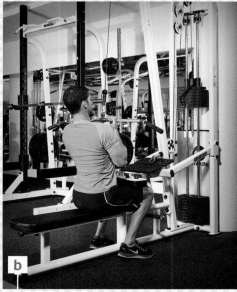

- Sit on the seat and take an underhand, shoulder-width grip on the bar.
- Looking forward, retract your shoulder blades and keep your torso upright.
- Pull the bar down in front of you until it reaches your upper chest. Don't lean back to aid the movement.
- Squeeze your lats at the bottom of the move and return the bar slowly to the top.

2 | Seated cable row

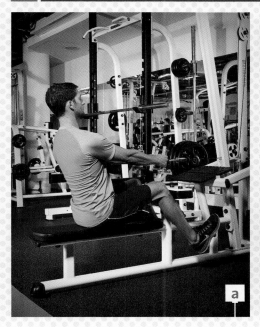
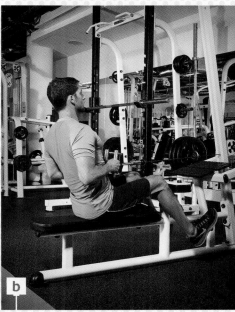

a

b

- Sit on the bench with a slight bend in your knees, holding a double-D handle – attached to the lower pulley of a cable machine – with a neutral grip.

- Make sure there is tension in the cable before you begin.

- Pull the handle in to your sternum, keeping upper-body movement to a minimum, and squeeze your shoulder blades together.

- Return slowly to the start.

TRAINER TIP

- Imagine someone has their finger in the middle of your upper back, and try to squash it with your shoulder blades.

3 | Reverse bench row

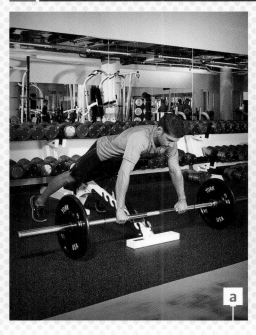
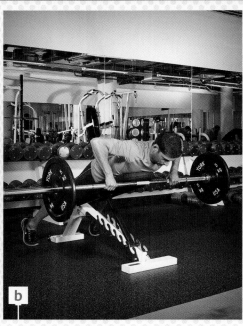

a

b

- Lie chest-first on an incline bench holding a barbell with a wide, overhand grip.

- Keeping your chest on the bench, shrug the barbell up, leading with your elbows.

- Return to the start.

TRAINER TIP

- Resist the temptation to use your arms. This is a back move so ensure that those muscles are behind the movement.

4 | Seated dumbbell shoulder press

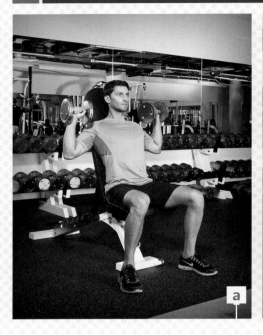
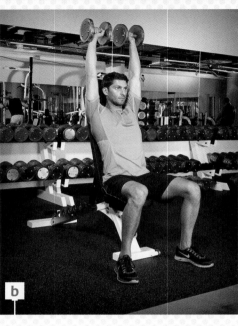

- Sit on an upright bench holding a dumbbell in each hand at shoulder height.
- Keep your feet flat on the floor, core braced, back against the bench and head looking forward.
- Press the weights up powerfully until your arms are fully extended, then return slowly to the start.

5 | Cable lateral raise

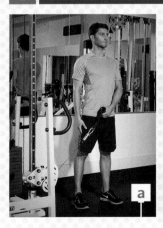
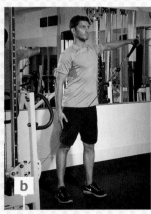

- Stand side-on to a cable machine holding a D-handle, attached to the low pulley, in your far hand.
- Keeping a slight bend in your elbows, lift your arm up and away from the machine. Stop at shoulder height, pause for a second and then slowly return to the start.
- Once you've completed all the reps, repeat with the other arm.

6 | Face pull

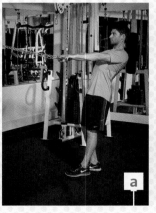
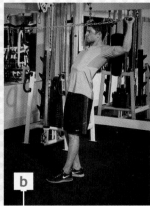

- Hold a double-rope attachment that's fixed to the high pulley on a cable machine.
- Start with arms fully extended and palms facing the floor.
- Pull the handles towards your head – keeping your upper arms parallel to the floor – so that the handles go to either side of your face.
- Return to the start.

Legs

EXERCISE	SETS	REPS	TEMPO	REST
SET 1				
1a Lying hamstring curl	2	6*	4010	30sec
1b Squat	2	12**	3010	60sec
SET 2				
2 Leg press	1	50	1010	120sec
SET 3				
3a Farmer's walk	4	40m	X	0sec
3b Reverse sled drag	4	40m	X	90–120sec
SET 4				
4a Decline plank with foot touch	4	24	2111	30sec
4b Garhammer raise	4	12	2010	60sec

* The final set is a drop set. Perform the stated number of reps, then reduce the weight by 15% and do them again. Repeat this process once more, then rest.

* * For the second set increase the weight so you reach failure at six reps. Reduce it again and perform six more reps, then again for six more, and then once more to complete this four-part set.

1a Lying hamstring curl

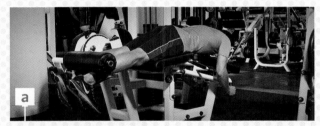

1b Squat

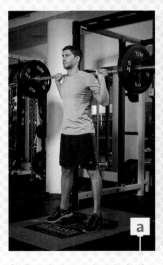
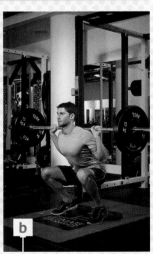

- Lie on the machine, following its instructions to position yourself correctly and safely.
- With the pad against the back of your lower calves, raise it up by contracting your hamstrings.
- Return slowly to the start.

- Rest the bar against the back of your shoulders – not your neck – and hold it with an overhand grip slightly wider than your shoulders. Keep your elbows pointing down.
- Your feet should be just wider than shoulder-width apart

with your toes pointing outwards slightly.
- Squat down until your thighs are at least parallel to the floor. The deeper you can squat, the better.
- Drive back up through your heels.

2 | Leg press

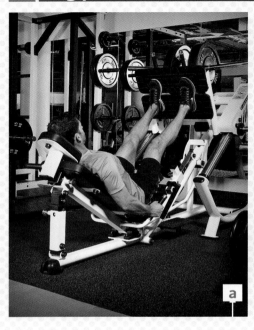
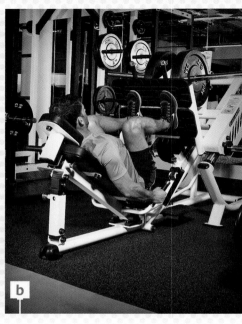

a b

- Sit on the machine, following its instructions to position yourself correctly and safely.
- Release the lock then slowly lower the platform towards you by bending your knees.
- Pause briefly at the bottom then push through your heels to straighten your legs and return to the start.

TRAINER TIP

- To get the most from this exercise, go up to 80% of full leg lock out. If you have to lock out, add five more reps to the set.

3a | Farmer's walk

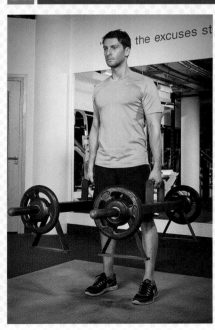

- Stand in front of a long, clear pathway holding a weighted bar or dumbbell in each hand.
- Keeping your core braced, walk as quickly as you can down the track.
- At the end, turn around and walk back quickly to the start.

3b | Reverse sled drag

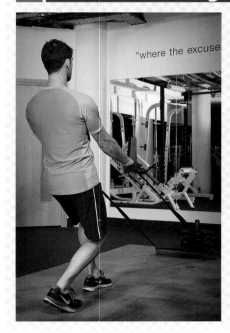

- Stand facing away from a long, clear pathway, holding a sled strap in each hand.
- Keeping your core braced and your arms straight, sprint backwards as fast as you can.
- At the end, turn around and sprint back to the start.

4a Decline plank with alternate foot touch

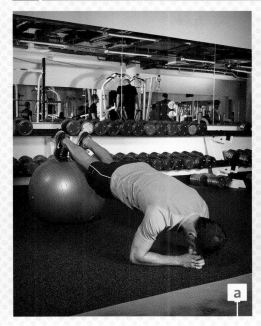
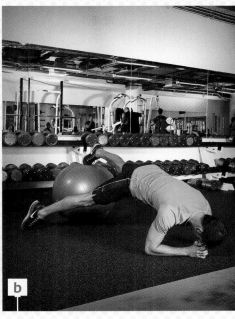

- With your feet on a raised platform, bench or gym ball, hold your body in a straight line from head to heels with your elbows beneath your shoulders and your head looking down.
- Hold the position and, without letting your hips sag, lift one foot up and out to the side, then lower it to the floor.
- Once you've touched the ground return that leg to the start position and repeat with your other leg.

4b Garhammer raise

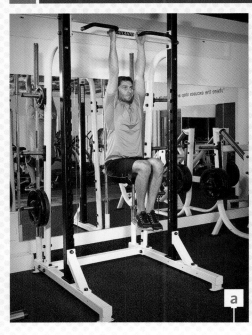
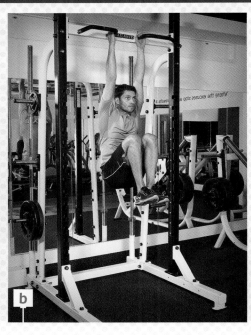

- Hang from a pull-up bar with your knees bent, then bring your knees in to your chest slightly so there is tension in your abs.
- Bring your knees further up towards your chest, maintaining the tension.
- Slowly lower them back down but only as far as the start position so that your abs never get the chance to relax from the strain of supporting your legs.

TRAINER TIP

- The point of this move is to keep your abs under tension. They should be starting to cramp up just before the set ends.

Chest and arms

EXERCISE	SETS	REPS	TEMPO	REST
SET 1				
1 Incline dumbbell bench press	2	10	3010	90sec
SET 2				
2 Incline dumbbell flye	2	12	3010	90sec
SET 3				
3 Pectoral dip	1	F*	4010	90sec
SET 4				
4a Spider curl	2	12	3011	60sec
4b Decline EZ-bar triceps extension	2	12	4010	60sec
SET 5				
5a Standing cable hammer curl	2	12**	3010	60sec
5b Incline EZ-bar triceps press	2	12+	4010	60sec
SET 6				
6 Diamond press-up	1	F*	3010	0sec

*
F means to failure. Once you reach failure, pause in the top position for 20sec and go again to failure. Repeat twice more.

**
The last set is a drop set. Perform the stated number of reps, then reduce the weight by 15% and do them again. Repeat the process once more, and rest.

+
After your final set of incline EZ-bar triceps presses, go straight into the diamond press-up to failure.

1 | Incline dumbbell bench press

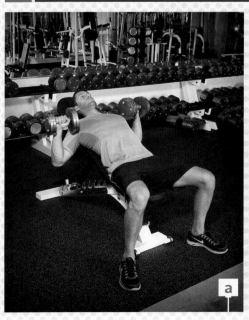
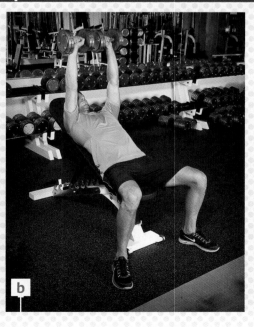

a

b

- Lie on a bench set at a 45° angle holding a dumbbell in each hand at shoulder-height.
- Keep your feet flat on the floor and your back against the bench.
- Press the weight directly above your head but don't lock out your elbows at the top.
- Slowly lower the weight back down to your chest, flaring your elbows out to the side.

2 | Incline dumbbell flye

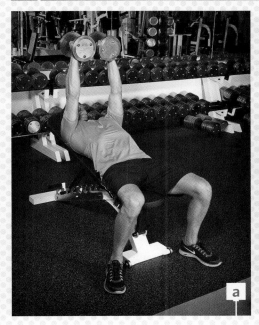
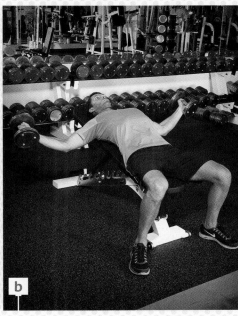

a   b

O Lie on an incline bench holding a dumbbell in each hand directly above your chest with palms facing.

O Make sure your head and upper back are supported on the bench and that your feet are flat on the floor.

O Keeping a slight bend in your elbows, slowly lower the weights out to the side as far as is comfortable.

O Use your chest to reverse the movement and raise the weights back to the top.

TRAINER TIP

O Use half the weight you think you can lift and concentrate on stretching, squeezing and opening your chest as much as possible.

3 | Pec dip

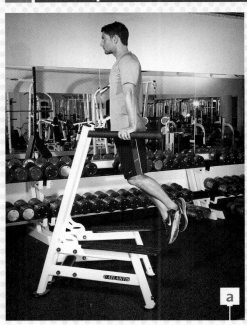
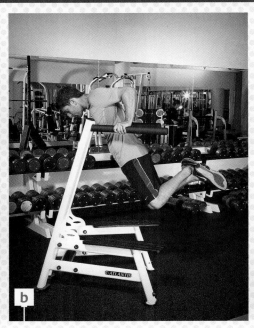

a   b

O Grip parallel bars and lean forward. Continue to lean forward throughout the move.

O With your elbows pointing straight back, lower your body as far as you can comfortably go without stressing your shoulders.

O Don't swing your legs for momentum.

O Press back up powerfully, focusing on contacting your chest muscles as hard as possible.

TRAINER TIP

O To get more out of this move, try to keep your chin pressed against your chest throughout.

4a Spider curl

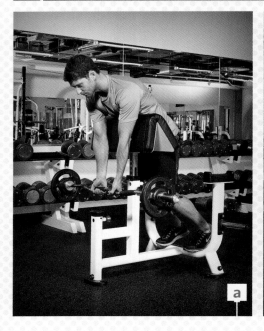
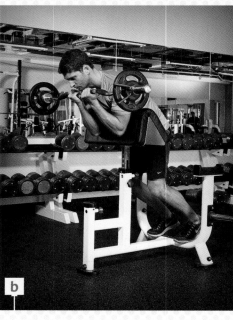

- Lean over a preacher bench with your chest flat against it and your arms fully extended holding an EZ-bar with a narrow grip.
- Curl the bar up to shoulder height, keeping your elbows against the padding.
- Slowly lower the bar back down for three seconds until your arms are fully straight, flexing your triceps at the bottom.

4b Decline EZ-bar triceps extension

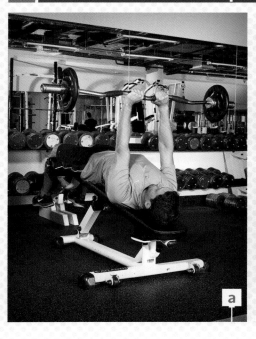
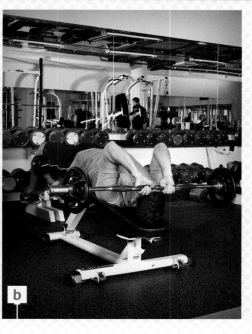

- Lie on a decline bench holding an EZ-bar above you with straight arms.
- Slowly lower the bar towards the top of your head by bending your elbows, which should point at the ceiling throughout.
- Without arching your back, slowly return the bar to the start position by straightening your arms.

5a Standing cable hammer curl

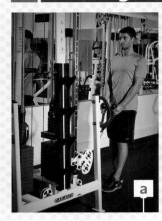
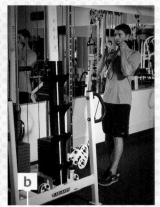

- Stand tall holding a double-rope cable handle, attached to the low pulley of a cable machine, with your palms facing each other.
- Keeping your elbows next to your body, curl your hands up to raise the handles towards your chin.
- Squeeze your biceps at the top of the move, then return to the start, squeezing your triceps and the very bottom.

5b Incline EZ-bar triceps press

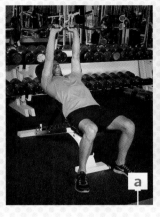
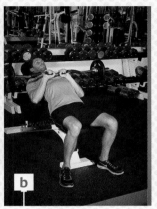

- Lie on a bench set at a 20° angle holding an EZ-bar with a narrow, overhand grip.
- Keep your feet flat on the floor and your back against the bench.
- Press the weight directly above your head but don't lock out your elbows at the top.
- Slowly lower the weight back down to your chest, keeping your elbows close to your side.

6 Diamond press-up

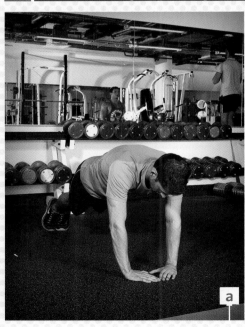
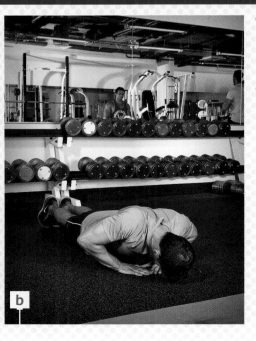

- Start in a press-up position but with your hands close together so that your thumbs and index fingers touch to form a diamond shape.
- Keeping your body in a straight line from head to heels, lower your chest as far as you can before powering back up strongly.

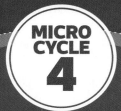

MICRO CYCLE 4

WORKOUTS
21 TO 29

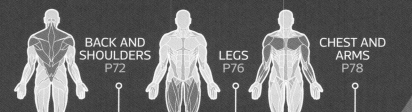

BACK AND
SHOULDERS
P72

LEGS
P76

CHEST AND
ARMS
P78

21 24 27   22 25 28   23 26 29

HEAVY METAL

Heavy weights and low reps keep your muscles guessing

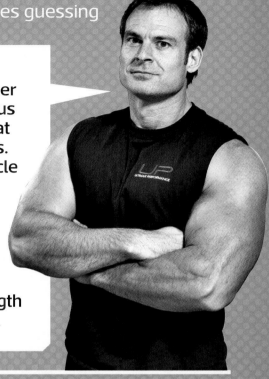

This microcycle shakes things up again with a return to a heavier phase of training, with bigger weights but lower reps. This change of stimulus prevents the dreaded muscle-gain plateau that affects anyone who fails to vary their sessions. Despite the low reps you can still expect muscle growth as there is a high degree of volume in these workouts, as well as more hardcore drop sets to work your muscles to fatigue.

The 25-rep drops sets are horrible but stick to the exact workouts I've created. And stay positive no matter how much it hurts: now is the time when you should be noticing strength gains as well as greater muscle development.

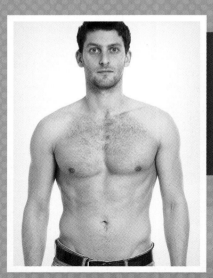

MICROCYCLE 4

WEIGHT
74.4kg

BODY FAT
PERCENTAGE
10.1%

HOW TO DO THESE WORKOUTS

Do workout 21 (back and shoulders), 22 (legs) and 23 (chest and arms) in order, before repeating this sequence with workouts 24 through to 29 then advancing to the next microcycle. Increase the weight for each session without losing form. Never work out on more than two consecutive days.

Back and shoulders

EXERCISE	SETS	REPS	TEMPO	REST
SET 1				
1a Rack deadlift	5	5	3111	90sec
1b Seated barbell shoulder press	5	5	4010	90sec
SET 2				
2a Reverse incline dumbbell row	4	6	3010	90sec
2b Dumbbell high pull	4	6	2010	90sec
SET 3				
3a Incline reverse dumbell flye	3	15	3010	0sec
3b Dumbbell shrug	3	15	2010	0sec
3c Face pull	3	15	2010	60sec

1a | Rack deadlift

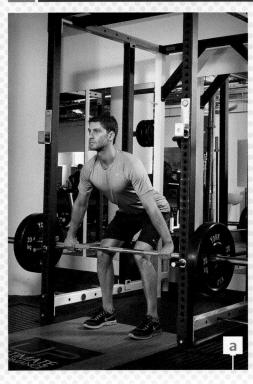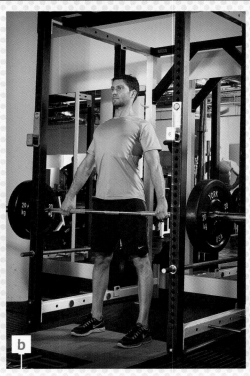

a

b

- Set the safety bars on a squat rack to mid-knee level.
- With the barbell resting on the bars, take a wide grip with your core braced, your back flat and your shoulders retracted and over the bar.
- Use your glutes to power the initial lift, pushing down through your heels.
- Keep the bar close to your body and, as it passes your knees, push your hips forward then lower the weight back down so it just touches the bars and repeat.

TRAINER TIP

- Stick your chest up and out at the top to contract your upper back muscles. Don't lean back with your lower back.

1b | Seated barbell shoulder press

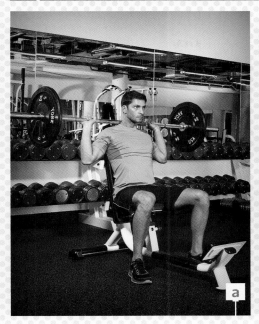
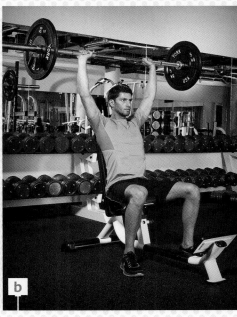

a
b

- Sit on an upright bench with a barbell on your upper chest, gripping it with hands shoulder-width apart.
- Keep your chest upright and your core muscles braced.
- Press the bar directly upwards until your arms are extended overhead.
- Lower the bar back down behind your neck then press back up.

2a | Reverse incline dumbbell row

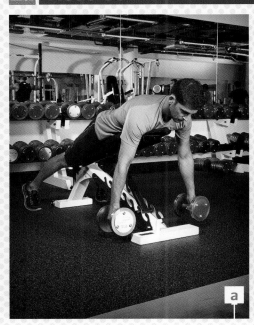
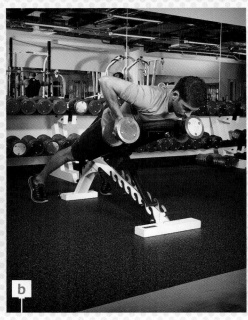

a
b

- Lie chest-first on an incline bench holding a dumbbell in each hand with your arms fully extended.
- Leading with your elbows, row the weights up towards you, focusing on retracting your shoulder blades rather than relying on your biceps.
- Slowly return to the start.

TRAINER TIP

- Maintain contact between the bench and your chest. If it's coming away from the bench the weight is too heavy.

2b Dumbbell high pull

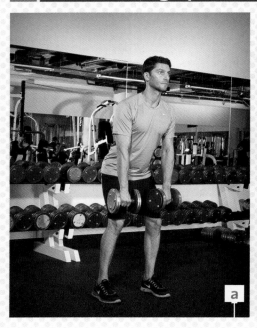
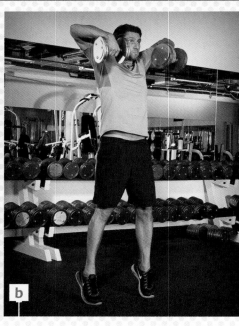

a | b

- Stand tall with a dumbbell in each hand with an overhand grip.
- Keeping your core braced, pull the weights up, leading with your elbow, until they are at chest height.
- Return to the start.

3a Incline reverse dumbbell flye

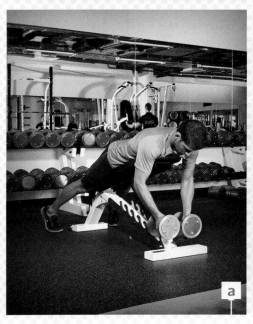
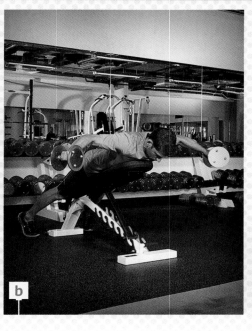

a | b

- Lie chest–forward on an incline bench holding a dumbbell in each hand.
- With a slight bend in your elbows, raise the weights out to your side until they reach shoulder height, then return to the start.

TRAINER TIP

- Don't go too heavy. Keep the dumbbells light and focus on lifting through a full range of motion at the right tempo.

3b Dumbbell shrug

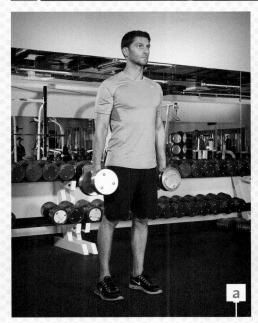
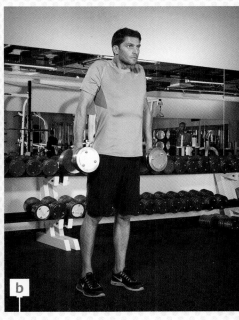

a   b

- Stand with two heavy dumbbells in front of you.
- Squat down and grip the weight securely with an overhand grip.
- Stand up, keeping your core braced and a natural arch in your back.
- Shrug your shoulders up towards your ears, keeping your arms straight.
- Hold for a second at the top position before slowly lowering the weight back down.

TRAINER TIP

- The limited range of motion allows you to go heavy here. Just deadlift the dumbbells safely to the start position.

3c Face pull

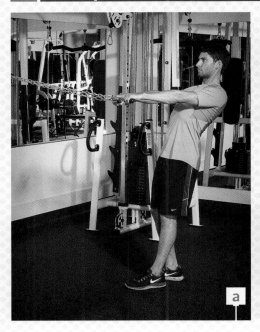
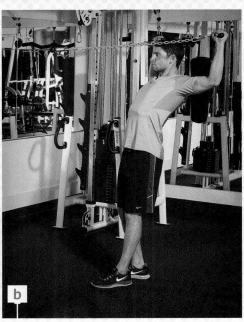

a   b

- Hold a double-rope attachment that's fixed to the high pulley on a cable machine.
- Start with your arms fully extended and your palms facing the floor.
- Pull the handles towards your head – keeping your upper arms parallel to the floor – so that the handles go to either side of your face.
- Return to the start.

Legs

EXERCISE	SETS	REPS	TEMPO	REST
SET 1				
1a Squat	6*	6	4010	150sec
1b Lying hamstring curl	6*	4	4011	120sec
SET 2				
2a **Reverse sled drag**	4	40m	X	0sec
2b **Dumbbell step-up**	4	15	2010	90sec

* After the final set, reduce the weight and perform 25 reps.

1a Squat

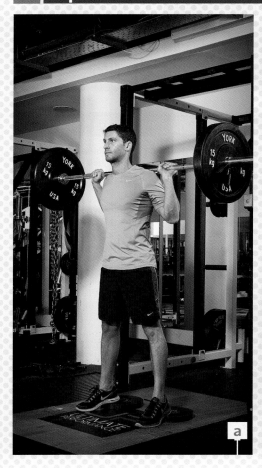
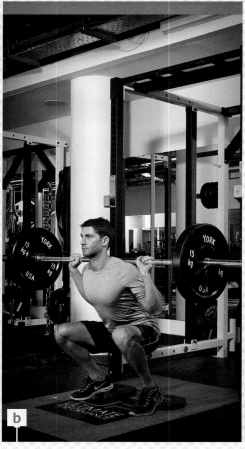

a   b

- Rest the bar against the back of your shoulders – not on your neck – and hold it with an overhand grip slightly wider than your shoulders. Keep your elbows pointing down.
- Your feet should be just wider than shoulder-width apart with your toes pointing outwards slightly.
- Squat down until your thighs are at least parallel to the floor. The deeper you can squat, the better.
- Drive back up through your heels.

TRAINER TIP

- With the extended drop set you really need a spotter on hand. If you can rope in two people to strip the weights for you, that will minimise the rest intervals.

1b Lying hamstring curl

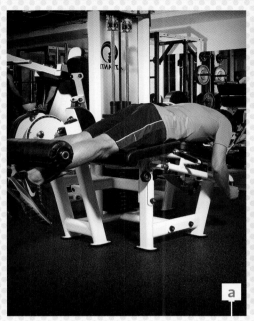
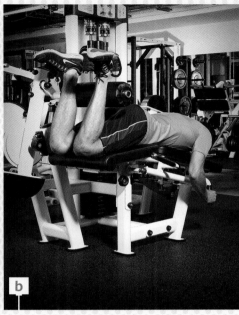

- Lie on the machine, following its instructions to position yourself correctly and safely.
- With the pad against the back of your lower calves, raise it by contracting your hamstrings.
- Return slowly to the start.

2a Reverse sled drag

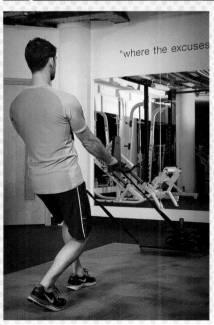

- Stand facing away from a long, clear pathway, holding a sled strap in each hand.
- Keeping your core braced and your arms straight, sprint backwards as fast as you can.
- At the end, turn around and sprint back to the start.

2b Dumbbell step-up

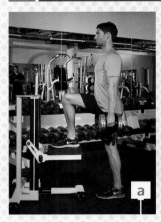

- Stand in front of a platform set at knee height holding a dumbbell in each hand.
- Keep one foot on the platform and step up and back down with the other.
- Switch legs and repeat.

Chest and arms

EXERCISE	SETS	REPS	TEMPO	REST
SET 1				
1a Incline bench press	5	5	4010	90sec
1b Chin-up	5	5	4010	90sec
SET 2				
2a Triceps dip	4	7	3010	75sec
2b Preacher dumbell hammer curl	4	7	3010	75sec
SET 3				
3a Barbell rollout	4	6	4010	60sec
3b Hanging leg raise	4	12	4010	90sec

1a | Incline bench press

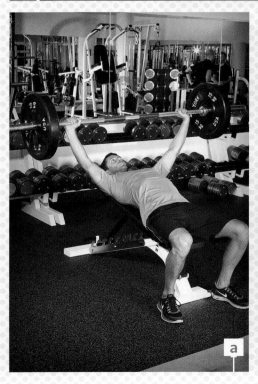
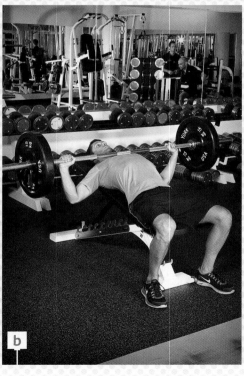

a

b

- Lie on a bench set at a **45°** angle holding a barbell with an overhand grip.
- Keep your feet flat on the floor and your back against the bench.
- Slowly lower the weight down to your chest, flaring your elbows out to the sides, until the bar touches your chest.
- Press the weight directly above your head but don't lock out your elbows at the top.

1b Chin-up

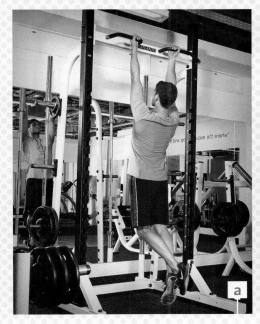
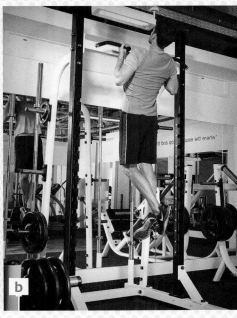

a

b

○ Grab the bar with an underhand grip with your hands slightly wider than shoulder-width apart.

○ Start from a dead hang with your arms fully extended.

○ Pull yourself up by squeezing your lats together.

○ Once your chin is higher than your hands lower yourself back to the start.

TRAINER TIP

○ You may need some additional weight for this move so use weight plates attached to a belt.

2a Triceps dip

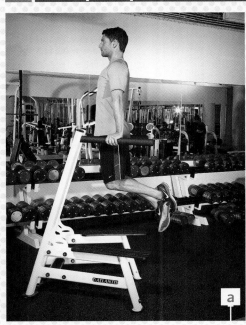
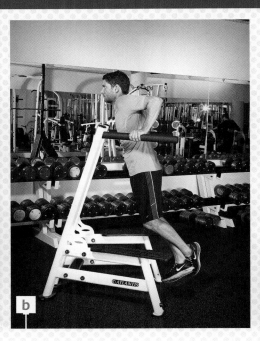

a

b

○ Grip parallel bars, keeping your body upright.

○ With your elbows pointing straight back, lower your body as far as you can comfortably go without stressing your shoulders.

○ Keep your core braced and don't swing your legs for momentum.

○ Press back up powerfully but don't lock out your elbows at the top.

TRAINER TIP

○ For additional weight you can always position a dumbbell between your feet.

2b Preacher dumbbell hammer curl

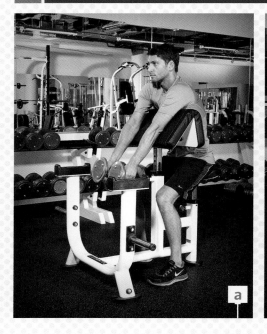
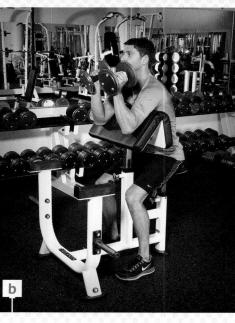

- Sit at a preacher bench holding a dumbbell in each hand with a neutral grip.
- Keeping your elbows on the bench, lift the dumbbells up towards your chin.
- Lower back slowly to the start.
- Avoid rocking back and forth to generate momentum, which takes the emphasis away from the biceps.

3a Barbell rollout

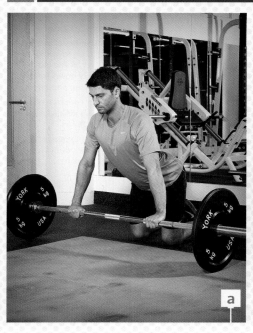
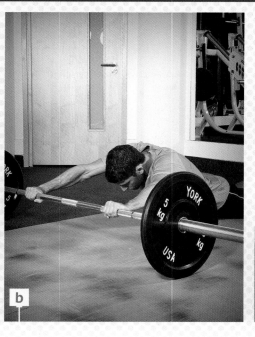

- Get on your knees with your arms extended and your hands holding a barbell with a shoulder-width grip.
- Slowly roll the barbell away from your body, keeping your core braced throughout.
- Once you have extended until your torso is parallel to the ground, contract your abs to pull the bar back towards your body.

TRAINER TIP

- You want your abs to be under tension for the entire set, so never return to a fully upright position.

3b | Hanging leg raise

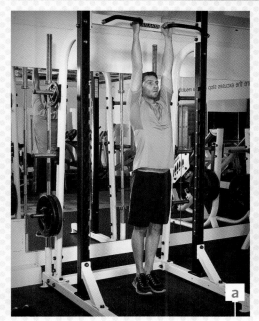
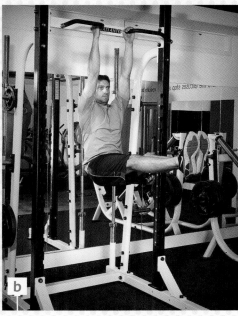

a b

- Hang from a bar with your body straight.
- Keeping your legs straight, use your lower abs to raise them until they are parallel with the ground.
- Return slowly to the start.

SPEED UP YOUR SIX-PACK
Now's the time to crank up your fat-loss efforts

By now you should have noticed some significant changes to your body. New muscles will have sprouted where there was none before, and your fat stores should be significantly reduced. However, if you're still not satisfied with the development of your six-pack, now is the time to introduce two types of cardio training to accelerate fat loss: high-intensity interval training and fasted walking. Don't worry if that sounds daunting – they are both incredibly simple to do and can make a huge difference in torching your remaining body fat. Turn to p134 for all the details on how and when to do these sessions, as well as our complete guide to carving an impressive six-pack so that you can start to process of putting the finishing touches to your physique. The chapter includes:

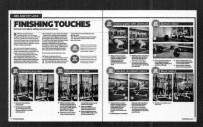

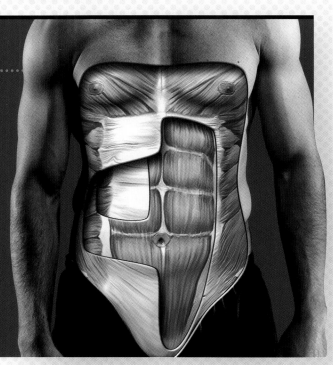

- Six-pack science: Nick answers the most common six-pack-related questions
- Finishing touches: the six best moves you can add to your workouts to carve a six-pack
- Blast away fat: clever cardio that will get you ripped

MICRO CYCLE 5

WORKOUTS
30 TO 38

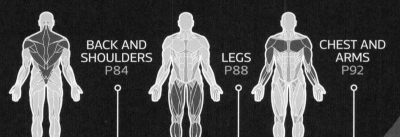

BACK AND SHOULDERS
P84

LEGS
P88

CHEST AND ARMS
P92

| 30 | 33 | 36 | 31 | 34 | 37 | 32 | 35 | 38 |

FEEL THE PUMP

These multi-move sets build muscle and burn fat

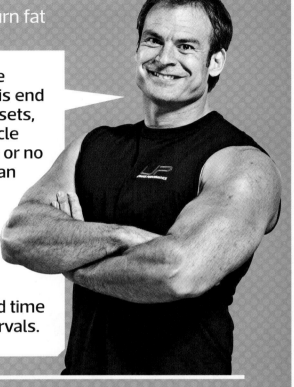

This microcycle maximises blood flow to the muscles to encourage greater returns. To this end there's a greater focus on tri-sets and giant sets, where multiple exercises for the same muscle group are performed back to back with little or no rest. This burns body fat more effectively than any extended cardio session, and creates extreme blood flow to the muscle.

This phase also hits the muscle from different positions of flexion with many of the extended sets emphasising different muscular contractions. Many of the sets are low-rep so you'll get the benefit of extended time under tension because of the short rest intervals.

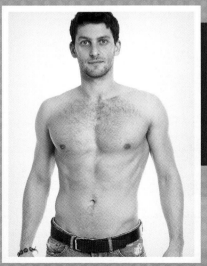

MICROCYCLE 5

WEIGHT
74.7kg

BODY FAT PERCENTAGE
8.7%

HOW TO DO THESE WORKOUTS

Do workout 30 (back and shoulders), 31 (legs) and 32 (chest and arms) in order, before repeating this sequence with workouts 33 through to 38 then advancing to the next microcycle. Increase the weight for each session without losing form. Never work out on more than two consecutive days.

Back and shoulders

EXERCISE	SETS	REPS	TEMPO	REST
SET 1				
1a Pull-up	3	6	4010	10sec
1b Dumbbell pull-over	3	8	3010	10sec
1c Seated cable row	3	8	3010	10sec
1d Rack deadlift	3	10	2111	120sec
SET 2				
2a Seated shoulder press	3	6	4010	0sec
2b Cable lateral raise	3	10	2010	0sec
2c Cable upright row	3	12	2010	90sec

1a Pull-up

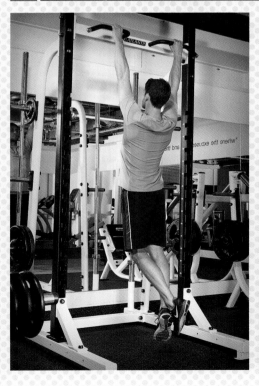
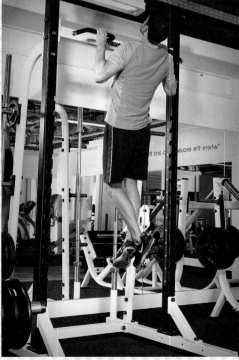

- Grab the bar with an overhand grip with your hands shoulder-width apart.
- Start from a dead hang with your arms fully extended.
- Pull yourself up by squeezing your lats together.
- Once your chin is higher than your hands pause briefly, then slowly lower yourself back to the start.

TRAINER TIP

- Keep your chest up throughout and don't allow the weight plates or dumbbells to swing if you are using them for extra resistance.

1b | Dumbbell pull-over

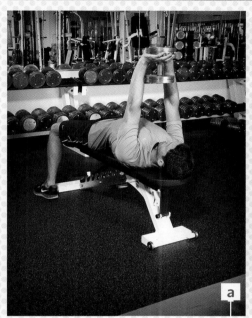
a

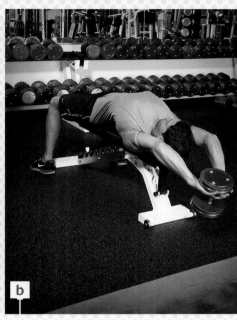
b

- Lie flat on a bench with your head and shoulders supported and your feet flat on the floor.
- Hold a single dumbbell over your chest with both hands and engage your core.
- Slowly lower the weight behind your head, keeping a slight bend in your elbows. Don't arch your back.
- Raise the weight back over your head to the start position.

TRAINER TIP

- We want this move to hit your back muscles so focus on lifting with only the muscles in your upper back.

1c | Seated cable row

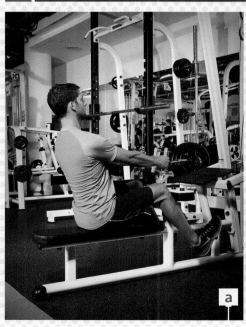
a

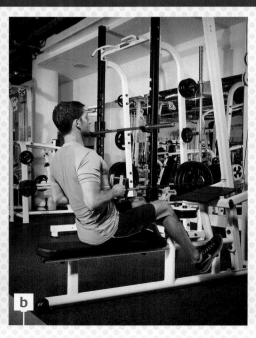
b

- Sit on the bench with a slight bend in your knees, holding a double-D handle – attached to the lower pulley of a cable machine – with a neutral grip.
- Make sure there is tension in the cable before you begin.
- Pull the handle in to your sternum, keeping upper-body movement to a minimum, and squeeze your shoulder blades together.
- Return slowly to the start.

1d | Rack deadlift

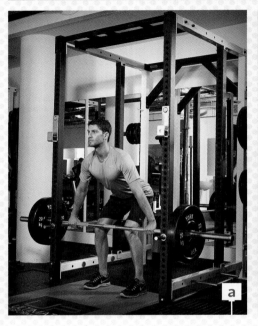
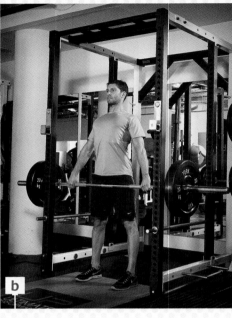

a

b

- Set the safety bars on a squat rack to mid-knee level.
- With the barbell resting on the bars, take a wide grip with your core braced, your back flat and your shoulders retracted and over the bar.
- Use your glutes to power the initial lift, pushing down through your heels.
- Keep the bar close to your body and, as it passes your knees, push your hips forward then lower the weight back down so it just touches the bars and repeat.

TRAINER TIP

- Really focus on squeezing your shoulder blades back and standing tall to hit the target muscles.

2a | Seated shoulder press

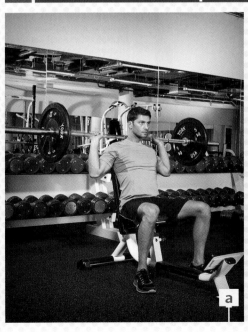
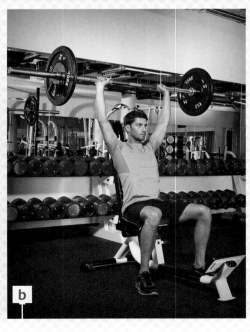

a

b

- Sit on an upright bench with a barbell on your upper chest, gripping it with hands shoulder-width apart.
- Keep your chest upright and your core muscles braced.
- Press the bar directly upwards until your arms are extended overhead.
- Lower the bar back down behind your neck then press back up.

2b Cable lateral raise

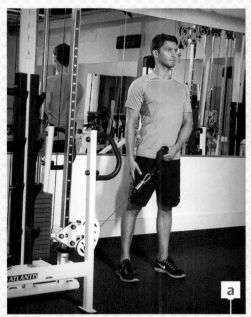
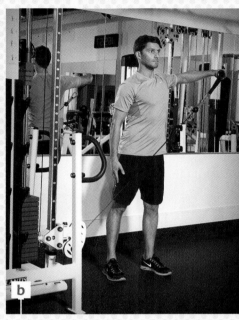

a
b

- Stand side-on to a cable machine holding a D-handle, attached to the low pulley, in your far hand.
- Keeping a slight bend in your elbows, lift your arm up and away from the machine. Stop at shoulder height then slowly return to the start.
- Once you've completed all the reps, repeat with the other arm.

TRAINER TIP

- Stand tall, avoiding any inclination to lean forward, and focus on your delts as they lift and lower the weight.

2c Cable upright row

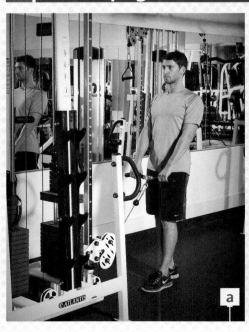
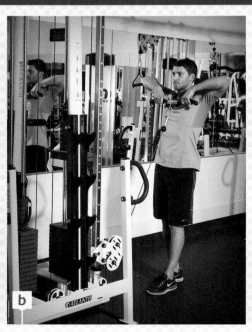

a
b

- Stand tall holding a straight or EZ-bar handle, attached to the low pulley of a cable machine, with an overhand grip.
- Leading with your elbows, pull the bar up until your hands are at shoulder-height.
- Slowly lower the bar back to the start.

Legs

EXERCISE	SETS	REPS	TEMPO	REST
SET 1				
1a Lying hamstring curl	4	6	3010	10sec
1b Weighted glute bridge	4	10	2011	0sec
1c Walking dumbbell lunge	4	40m	x	90sec
SET 2				
2a Front squat*	10	6	3010	0sec
2b Squat	10	9	3010	60sec
SET 3				
3a Barbell rollout	4	6	4010	0sec
3b Hanging leg raise	4	12	4010	30sec
3c Decline dumbbell crunch	4	12	2010	60sec

* The aim is to complete all ten sets of front squats and squats within 25 minutes.

1a | Lying hamstring curl

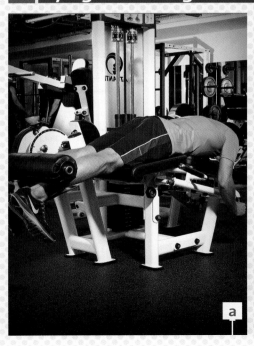
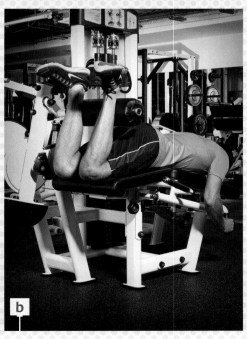

a   b

- Lie on the machine, following its instructions to position yourself correctly and safely.
- With the pad against the back of your lower calves, raise it up by contracting your hamstrings.
- Return slowly to the start.

1b | Weighted glute bridge

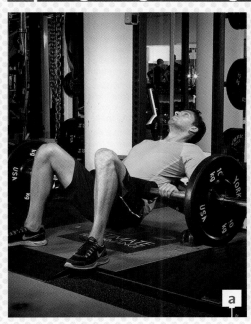

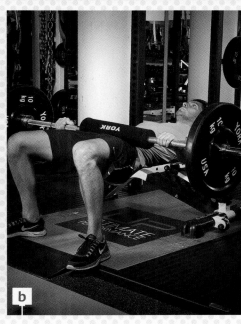

a

b

- Lie with your upper back supported on a bench, your feet flat on the floor and your knees bent, with a barbell resting across your hips.
- Squeeze your glutes to lift the weight and return to the start position.
- Brace your core and lower your glutes down towards the floor.

1c | Walking dumbbell lunge

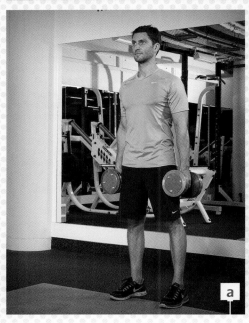

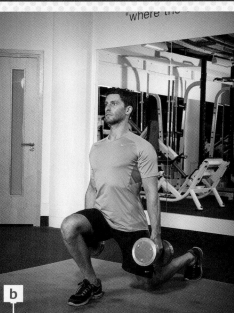

a

b

- Stand in front of a long, clear pathway, holding a dumbbell in each hand.
- Keeping your core braced, take a big step forward and lunge down until both knees are bent at 90°.
- Push off from your back foot and lunge forward with that leg.
- Repeat until you have covered the stated distance.

TRAINER TIP

- A steady rhythm is key. You will want to stop, but ignore the pain, fix your eyes on the end point and keep moving.

2a Front squat

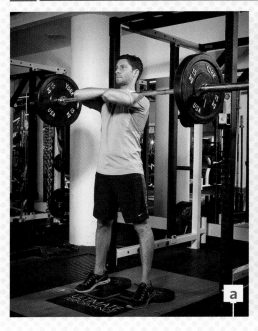
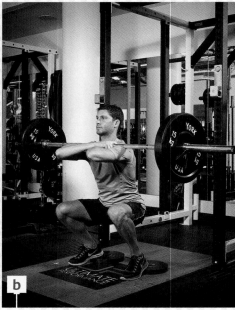

a b

- Rest the bar on the front of your shoulders, gripping it with your hands crossed in front of you, with your elbows pointing forward and feet shoulder-width apart.
- Maintain a natural arch in your back and keep your core braced throughout the move.
- Squat down until your thighs are at least parallel to the floor. The deeper you can squat, the better.
- Drive back up through your heels.

TRAINER TIPS

- Keep your elbows high. If they slip, your torso will follow and you'll be fighting the weight in the wrong direction.

2b Squat

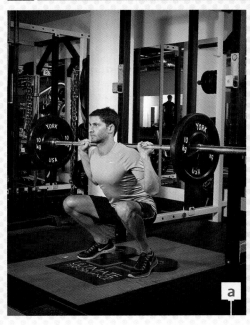
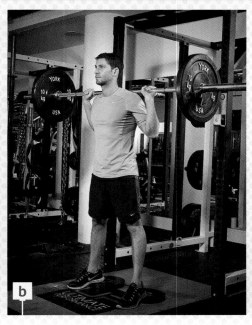

a b

- Rest the bar against the back of your shoulders – not on your neck – and hold it with an overhand grip slightly wider than your shoulders. Keep your elbows pointing down.
- Your feet should be just wider than shoulder-width apart with your toes pointing outwards slightly.
- Squat down until your thighs are at least parallel to the floor. The deeper you can squat, the better.
- Drive back up through your heels.

TRAINER TIPS

- At times during this superset you'll wonder why the hell you're doing this. Keep your overall goal in mind.

3a Barbell rollout

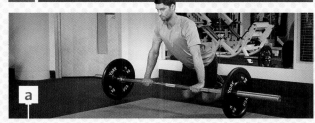

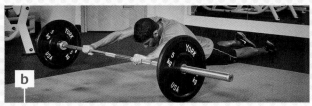

- Get on your knees with your arms extended and your hands holding a barbell with a shoulder–width grip.
- Slowly roll the barbell away from your body, keeping your core braced throughout.
- Once your have extended until your torso is parallel to the ground, contract your abs to pull the bar back towards your body to the start position.

3b Hanging leg raise

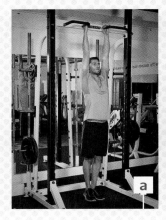
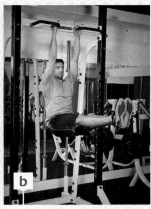

- Hang from a bar with your body straight.
- Keeping your legs straight, use your lower abs to raise them until they are parallel with the ground.

3c Decline dumbbell crunch

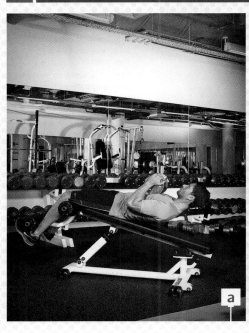
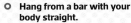
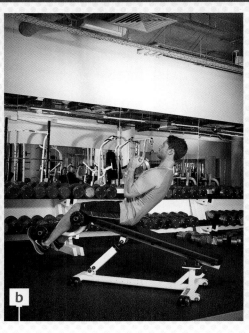

- Lie on a decline bench holding a dumbbell on your chest.
- Contract your abs to lift your shoulders up and curl your chest towards your knees.
- Pause at the top of the move, squeeze your abs and lower slowly to the start.

Chest and arms

EXERCISE	SETS	REPS	TEMPO	REST
SET 1				
1a Incline dumbbell bench press	3	6	3110	10sec
1b Decline bench press	3	6	4010	10sec
1c Dumbbell bench press	3	6	4010	90sec
SET 2				
2a EZ-bar preacher curl	3	6	4010	10sec
2b Incline dumbbell curl	3	6	3110	10sec
2c Kneeling overhead cable curl	3	6	3011	10sec
2d Triceps dip	3	6	4010	10sec
2e Decline lying triceps extension	3	6	4010	10sec
2f Standing overhead triceps extension	3	6	3110	45sec

1a | Incline dumbbell bench press

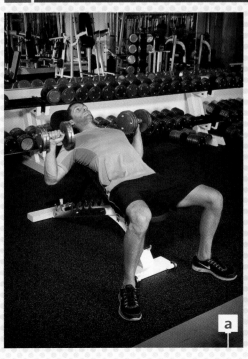
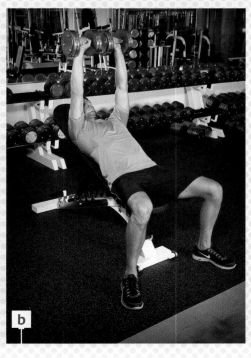

- Lie on a bench set at a 45° angle holding a dumbbell in each hand at shoulder-height.
- Keep your feet flat on the floor and your back against the bench.
- Press the weights directly above your head but don't lock out your elbows at the top.
- Slowly lower the weights back down to your chest, flaring your elbows out to the side.

1b | Decline bench press

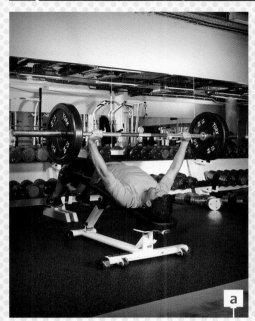 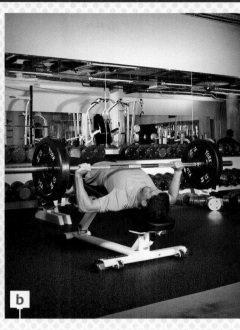

a   b

- Lie on a decline bench with your feet on the floor, directly under your knees.
- Hold the bar with an overhand grip shoulder–width apart.
- Slowly lower the bar to your chest, taking your elbows out to 90°, until the bar is almost touching the middle of chest or just over your nipples.
- Drive your feet hard into the floor and push the bar back strongly to the start position.

1c | Dumbbell bench press

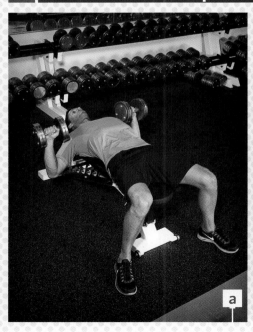 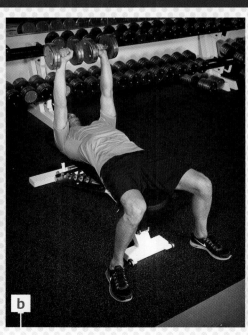

a   b

- Lie on a flat bench holding a dumbbell in each hand at shoulder–height.
- Keep your feet flat on the floor and your back against the bench.
- Press the weight directly above your head but don't lock out your elbows at the top.
- Slowly lower the weight back down to your chest, flaring your elbows out to the side.

TRAINER TIP

- You may be tempted not to stretch at the bottom of the move or contract hard at the top, but for maximum gains each rep must be perfect.

2a | EZ-bar preacher curl

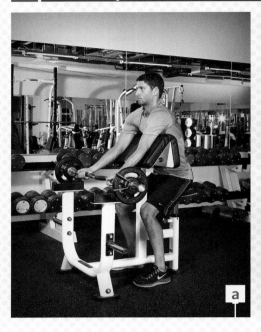
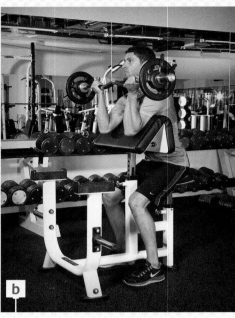

a b

- Sit at a preacher bench holding an EZ-bar with an overhand grip.
- Keeping your elbows on the bench, curl the bar up towards your chin.
- Lower back slowly to the start.
- Avoid rocking back and forth to generate momentum, which takes the emphasis away from the biceps.

2b | Incline dumbbell curl

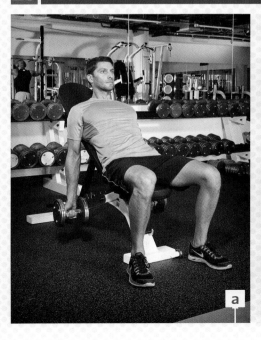
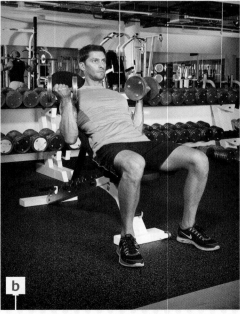

a b

- Sit on a bench set at an incline of between 30° and 45° holding a dumbbell in each hand.
- Keeping your back flat against the bench and your elbows close to your sides, slowly curl both dumbbells up to shoulder height.
- Squeeze your biceps at the top of the move before slowly returning to the start.

TRAINER TIP

- Squeeze your biceps at the top, flex your triceps at the bottom and cock your wrists back so you don't use your forearms.

2c Kneeling overhead cable curl

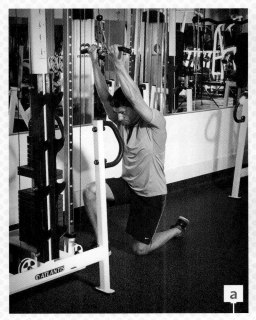
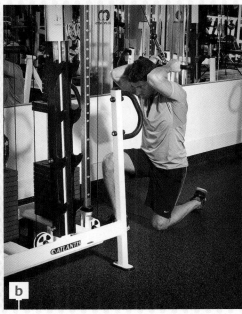

- Kneel in front of a cable machine holding an EZ–bar handle attached to a high cable.
- Keeping your elbows locked in position, curl the bar back behind your head.
- Return to the start.

2d Triceps dip

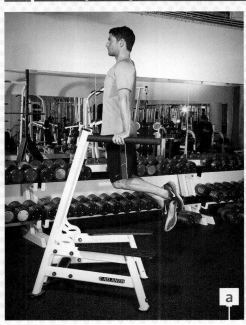
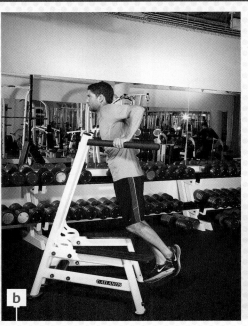

- Grip parallel bars, keeping your body upright.
- With your elbows pointing straight back, lower your body as far as you can comfortably go without stressing your shoulders.
- Keep your core braced and don't swing your legs for momentum.
- Press back up powerfully but don't lock out your elbows at the top.

TRAINER TIP

- If you can't complete all the reps, jump to the top position, lower yourself by 10cm and hold for as long as you can. Repeat three more times.

2e Decline lying triceps extension

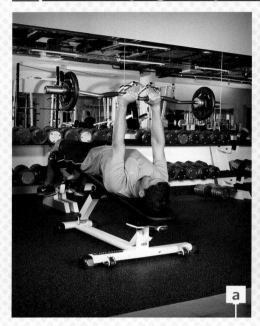
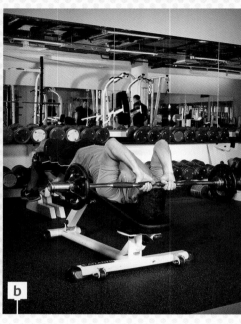

- Lie on a decline bench, holding an EZ-bar above you with straight arms.
- Slowly lower the bar towards the top of your head by bending your elbows, which should point at the ceiling throughout.
- Without arching your back, slowly return the bar to the start position by straightening your arms.

2f Standing overhead triceps extension

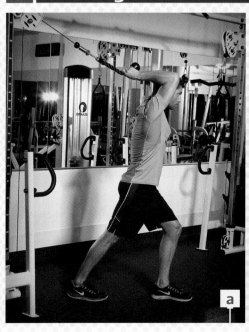
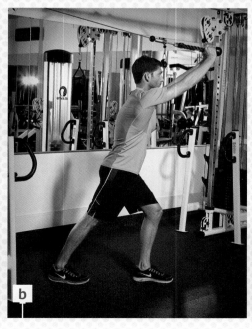

- Stand tall holding a double-rope handle attached to the low pulley of a cable machine.
- Turn away from the machine with your hands behind your head and your elbows at either side.
- Keeping your elbows next to your head, press the handles up and forward to straighten your arms.
- Flex your triceps at the top of the move, then return to the start and flex your biceps.

TRAINER TIP

- Resist the temptation to make things easier by letting your elbows flare out. Tuck them in tightly to get a greater stretch.

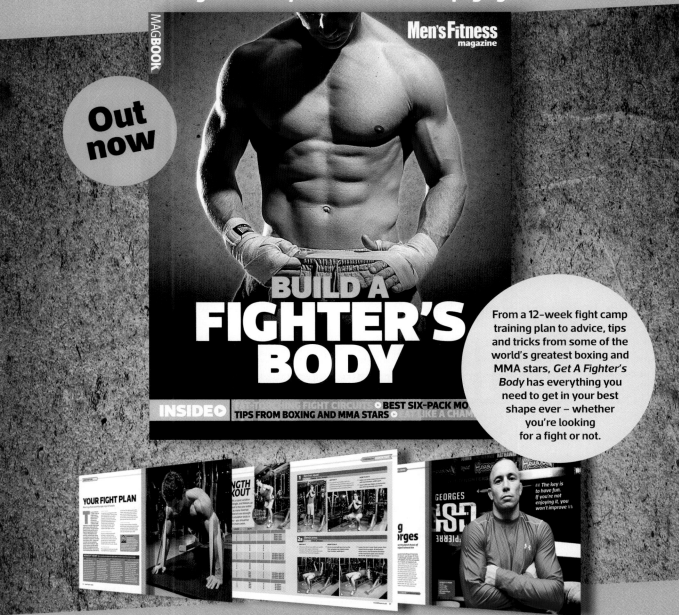

WORKOUTS
39 TO 41

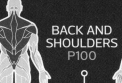

BACK AND
SHOULDERS
P100

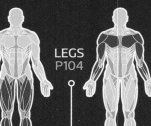

LEGS
P104

CHEST AND
ARMS
P108

39 40 41

KEEP ON GROWING

By now you've made real gains – but it's no time to slack off

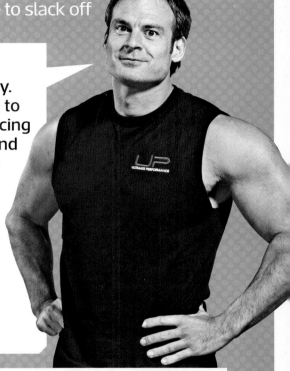

This short microcycle will provide a 'deload' as well as a short, sharp shock of training intensity. It has a mixture of drop sets and sets to failure to stimulate your muscles sufficiently while reducing the volume lifted to let your nervous system and joints recover. With most of the sessions in the bag, you should be noticing big differences in your physique and it may be tempting to take your foot of the gas a little. That's the wrong attitude. It's imperative that you step up the effort and execute each rep with total focus. Do that and your results will rocket.

Before starting this cycle, read the Finishing Touches chapter (p142) to ensure you look as good as possible when the training is over.

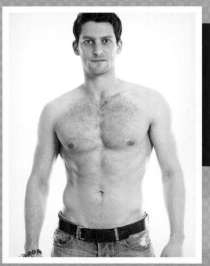

MICROCYCLE 6

WEIGHT
74.9kg

BODY FAT PERCENTAGE
7.8%

HOW TO DO THESE WORKOUTS

Read the Finishing Touches chapter on p142 then do workout 39 (back and shoulders), 40 (legs) and 41 (chest and arms) in order, before advancing to the next microcycle. Never work out on more than two consecutive days.

Back and shoulders

EXERCISE	SETS	REPS	TEMPO	REST
SET 1				
1a Lat pull-down	2	10	4010	90sec
1b Seated cable row	2*	10	3010	90sec
SET 2				
2a Reverse bench row	1*	10	3010	0sec
2b Seated dumbbell shoulder press	1	15	3010	30sec
SET 3				
3a Cable lateral raise	2*	12	3010	0sec
3b Face pull	2*	12	3010	30sec
SET 4				
4 Barbell rollout	2	8	4010	60sec

*
The final set is a drop set. Perform the stated number of reps, then reduce the weight by 15% and do the same number of reps. Repeat this process once more, then rest.

1a Lat pull-down

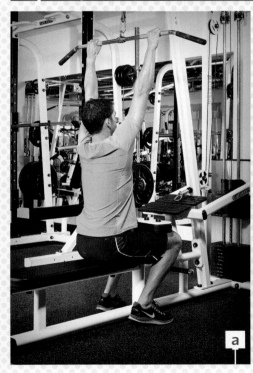
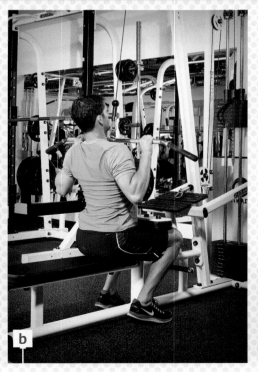

a   b

- Sit on the seat and hold the bar with an overhand, shoulder-width grip.
- Look forward, retract your shoulder blades and keep your torso upright.
- Pull the bar down in front of you until it reaches your upper chest. Don't lean back to aid the movement.
- Squeeze your lats at the bottom of the move and return the bar slowly to the top.

TRAINER TIP
- To engage your back rather than your biceps, drive your elbows back hard instead of pulling with your arms.

1b | Seated cable row

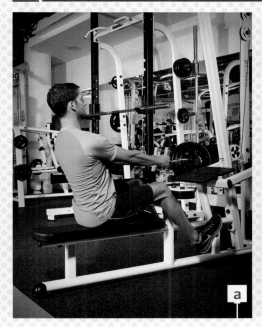
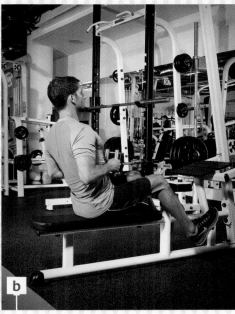

a   b

- Sit on the bench with a slight bend in your knees, holding a double-D handle – attached to the lower pulley of a cable machine – with a neutral grip .
- Make sure there is tension in the cable before you begin.
- Pull the handle in to your sternum, keeping upper-body movement to a minimum, and squeeze your shoulder blades together.
- Return slowly to the start.

2a | Reverse bench row

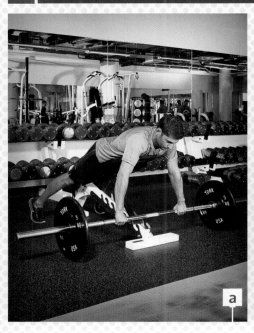
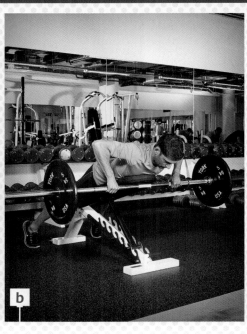

a   b

- Lie chest-first on an incline bench holding a barbell with a wide, overhand grip.
- Keeping your chest on the bench, row the barbell up, leading with your elbows.
- Return to the start.

2b Seated dumbbell shoulder press

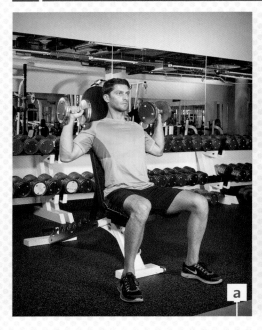

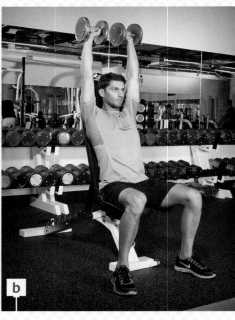

- Sit on an upright bench holding a dumbbell in each hand at shoulder height.
- Keep your feet flat on the floor, your core braced, your back against the bench and your head looking forward.
- Press the weights up powerfully until your arms are fully extended, then return slowly to the start.

3a Cable lateral raise

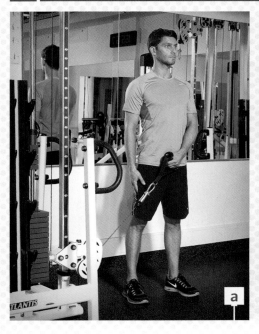

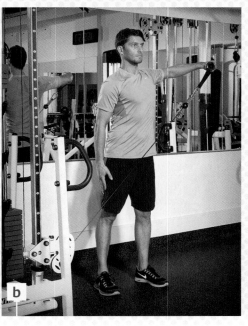

- Stand side-on to a cable machine holding a D-handle, attached to the low pulley, in your far hand.
- Keeping a slight bend in your elbows, lift your arm up and away from the machine. Stop at shoulder height, pause for a second and slowly return to the start.
- Once you've completed all the reps, repeat with the other arm.

3b Face pull

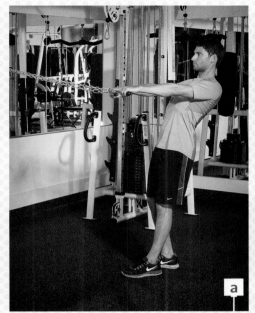
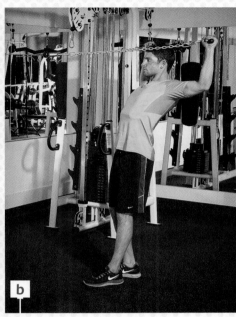

a

b

- Hold a double-rope attachment that's fixed to the high pulley on a cable machine.
- Start with arms fully extended and palms facing the floor.
- Pull the handles towards your head – keeping your upper arms parallel to the floor – so that the handles go to either side of your face.
- Return to the start.

TRAINER TIP

- If balance is an issue stand with a split-stance with one foot slightly in front of the other and brace your core.

4 Barbell rollout

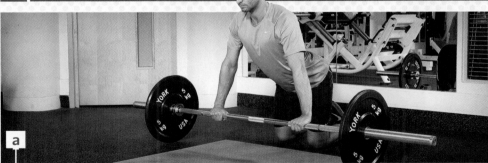

a

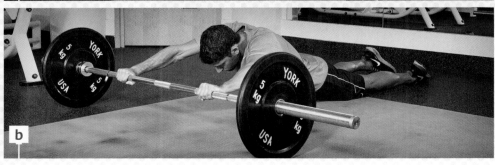

b

- Get on your knees with your arms extended and your hands holding a barbell with a shoulder-width grip.
- Slowly roll the barbell away from your body, keeping your core braced throughout.
- Once you have extended until your torso is parallel to the ground, contract your abs to pull the bar back towards your body to the start position.

Legs

EXERCISE	SETS	REPS	TEMPO	REST
SET 1				
1a Lying hamstring curl	2*	6	4010	90sec
1b Squat	2*	12	3010	120sec
SET 2				
2 Leg press	1	50	1010	180sec
SET 3				
3a Farmer's walk	4	30m	X	0sec
3b Reverse sled drag	4	30m	X	180sec
SET 4				
4a Decline dumbbell crunch	4	12	3010	30sec
4b Toes to bar	4	10	3010	0sec
4c Hanging leg raise	4	10	3010	60sec

 * Every set is to failure. Once you've performed the stated number of reps, reduce the weight by 15% and lift to failure, then lower the weight by a further 15% and do one more set to failure.

1a Lying hamstring curl

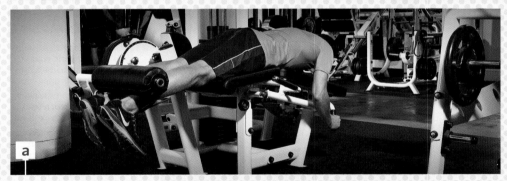

- Lie on the machine, following its instructions to position yourself correctly and safely.
- With the pad against the back of your lower calves, raise it up by contracting your hamstrings.
- Return slowly to the start.

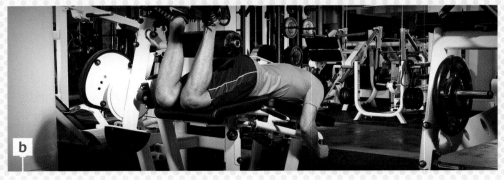

1b Squat

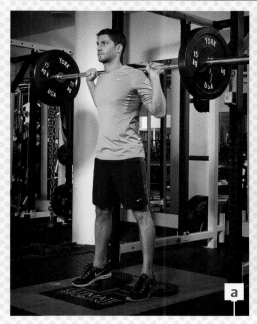
a

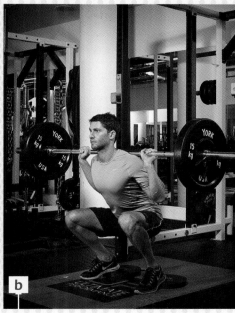
b

- Rest the bar against the back of your shoulders – not on your neck – and hold it with an overhand grip slightly wider than your shoulders. Keep your elbows pointing down.
- Your feet should be just wider than shoulder–width apart with your toes pointing outwards slightly.
- Squat down until your thighs are at least parallel to the floor. The deeper you can squat, the better.
- Drive back up through your heels.

2 Leg press

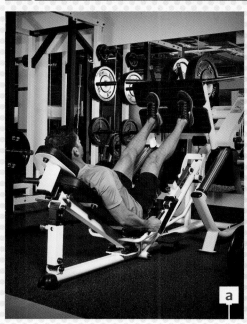
a

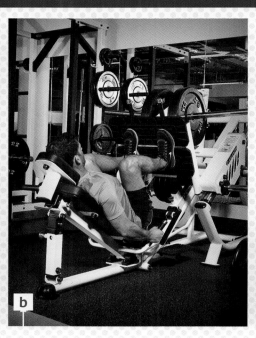
b

- Sit on the machine, following its instructions to position yourself correctly and safely.
- Release the lock then slowly lower the platform towards you by bending your knees.
- Push through your heels to straighten your legs and return to the start.

TRAINER TIP

- This is a 50–rep set, so don't lock out your legs completely. Maintain tension on your muscles throughout the set.

3a Farmer's walk

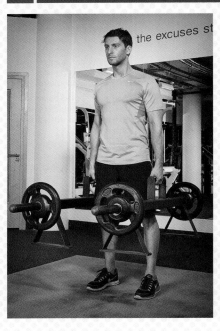

- Stand in front of a long, clear pathway, holding a weighted bar or dumbbell in each hand.
- Keeping your core braced, walk as quickly as you can down the track.
- At the end, turn around and walk back quickly to the start.

3b Reverse sled drag

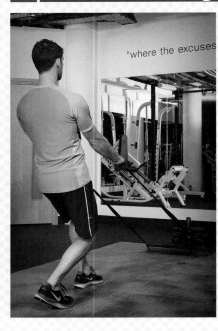

- Stand facing away from a long, clear pathway, holding a sled strap in each hand.
- Keeping your core braced and your arms straight, sprint backwards as fast as you can.
- At the end, turn around and sprint back to the start.

4a Decline dumbbell crunch

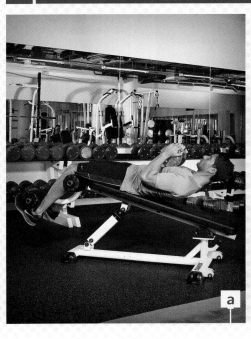
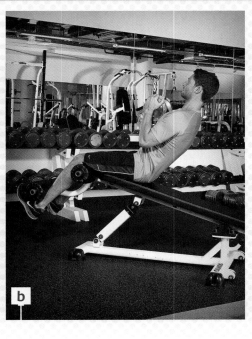

a   b

- Lie on a decline bench holding a dumbbell on your chest.
- Contract your abs to lift your shoulders up and curl your chest towards your knees.
- Pause at the top of the move, squeeze your abs then lower slowly to the start.

4b Toes to bar

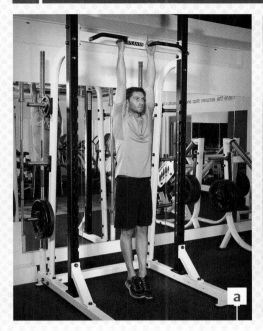 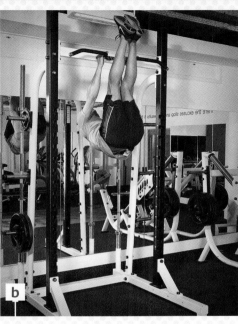

a

b

- Hang from a bar with your body straight.
- Keeping your legs as straight as possible, use your lower abs to lift them all the way up to the bar.
- Slowly lower them back to the start.

4c Hanging leg raise

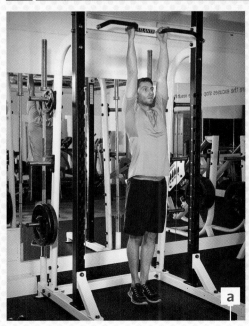 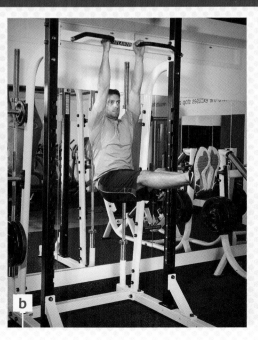

a

b

- Hang from a bar with your body straight.
- Keeping your legs straight, use your lower abs to raise them until they are parallel with the ground.

Chest and arms

EXERCISE	SETS	REPS	TEMPO	REST
SET 1				
1a Incline bench press	2	10	3010	30sec
1b Inline dumbbell flye	2	12	3010	30sec
SET 2				
2 Triceps dip	1	F*	4010	90sec
SET 3				
3a Spider curl	2	12	3011	0sec
3b Decline triceps extension	2	12	4010	90sec
SET 4				
4a Standing cable hammer curl	2	12+	3010	0sec
4b Incline EZ-bar triceps press	2	12**	4010	0sec
SET 5				
5 Diamond press-up	1	F*	2010	90sec

✱
F means to failure. Once you reach failure, pause in the top position for 20sec and go again to failure. Repeat twice more.

+
In the final set, perform the stated reps, then reduce the weight by 15% and repeat. Do the same again and rest.

✱✱
After your final set go straight into Set 5 without resting.

1 | Incline bench press

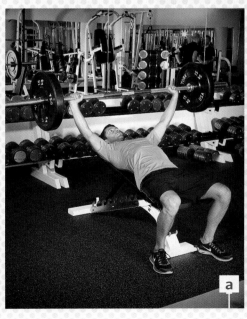
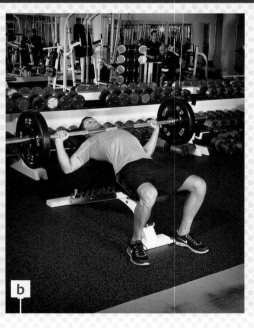

- Lie on an incline bench with your feet on the floor, directly under your knees.
- Hold the bar with an overhand grip shoulder-width apart.
- Slowly lower the bar to your chest, taking your elbows out to 90°, until the bar is almost touching the middle of your chest or just over your nipples.
- Drive your feet hard into the floor and push the bar back strongly to the start position.

1b Incline dumbbell flye

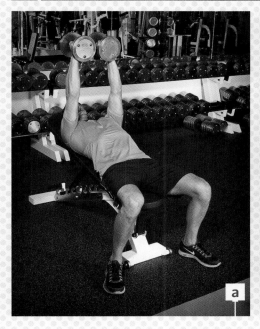

a

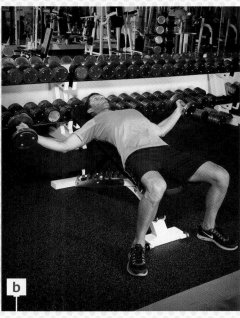

b

- Lie on an incline bench holding a dumbbell in each hand directly above your chest with palms facing.
- Make sure your head and upper back are supported on the bench and that your feet are flat on the floor.
- Keeping a slight bend in your elbows, slowly lower the weights out to the side as far as is comfortable.
- Use your chest to reverse the movement and raise the weights back to the top.

2 Triceps dip

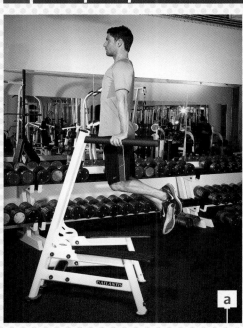

a

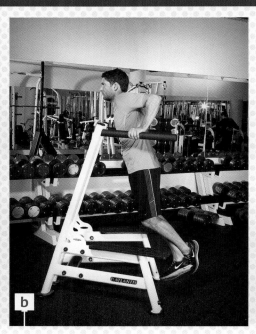

b

- Grip parallel bars, keeping your body upright.
- With your elbows pointing straight back, lower your body as far as you can comfortably go without stressing your shoulders.
- Keep your core braced and don't swing your legs for momentum.
- Press back up powerfully but don't lock out your elbows at the top.

TRAINER TIP

- It can be hard to stick to a tempo when nearing failure, but it's better to do quality reps than a few extra bad ones.

3a Spider curl

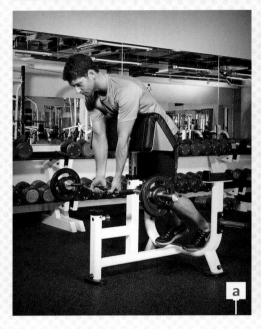
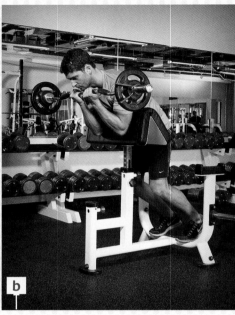

O Lean over a preacher bench with your chest flat against it and your arms fully extended holding an EZ-bar with a narrow grip.

O Curl the bar up to shoulder height, keeping your elbows against the padding.

O Slowly lower the bar back down in three seconds until your arms are straight, then flex your triceps at the bottom.

3b Decline EZ-bar triceps extension

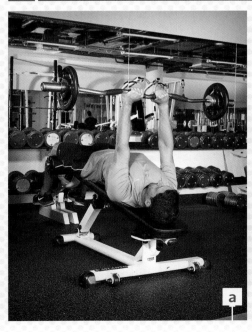
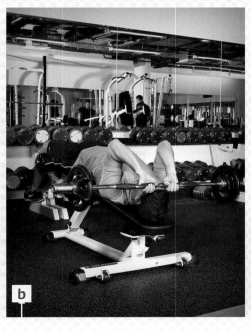

O Lie on a decline bench, holding an EZ-bar above you with straight arms.

O Slowly lower the bar towards the top of your head by bending your elbows, which should point at the ceiling throughout.

O Without arching your back, slowly return the bar to the start position by straightening your arms.

TRAINER TIP

O Keep your elbows pointing up throughout every rep to make sure the tension is solely on your triceps.

4a Standing cable hammer curl

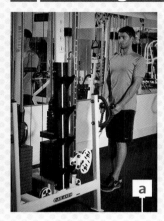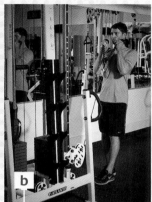

- Stand tall holding a double-rope cable handle, attached to the low pulley of a cable machine, with your palms facing each other.
- Keeping your elbows next to your body, curl your hands up to raise the handles

- towards your chin.
- Squeeze your biceps at the top of the move, then return to the start, flexing your triceps at the very bottom.

4b Incline EZ-bar triceps press

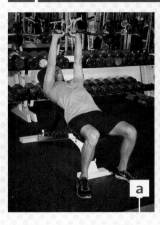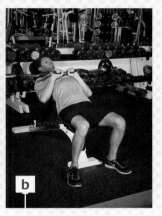

- Lie on a bench set at a 20° angle holding an EZ-bar with a narrow, overhand grip.
- Keep your feet flat on the floor and your back against the bench.
- Press the weight directly above your head but don't

- lock out your elbows at the top.
- Slowly lower the weight back down to your chest, keeping your elbows close to your side.

5 Diamond press-up

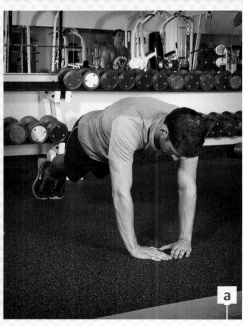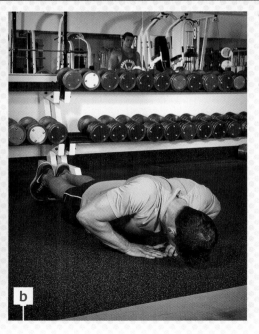

- Start in a press-up position but with your hands close together so that your thumbs and index fingers touch to form a diamond shape.
- Keeping your body in a straight line from head to heels, lower your chest as far as you can before powering back up strongly.

WORKOUTS 42 TO 44

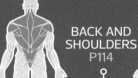

BACK AND SHOULDERS
P114

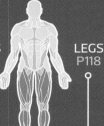

LEGS
P118

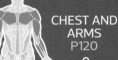

CHEST AND ARMS
P120

42 43 44

STRONG FINISH

With most of the work done, it's time for some fine-tuning

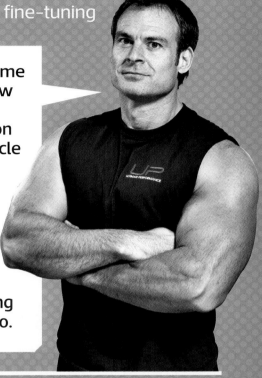

Congratulations! If you've stuck to the programme your muscles will ache in places you didn't know you had muscles and you'll be very bored with your diet, but you're close to being in possession of a brand new body. This penultimate microcycle is about putting the finishing touches to your physique, so you need to stay focused.

With 41 gruelling sessions in the bag, you're probably tired, so it may be time to reduce the workout intensity and prevent overtraining. If you still feel relatively good, by all means push harder by adding a drop-set to each exercise. But if you've been following everything perfectly, you shouldn't really want or be able to.

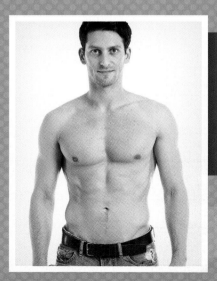

MICROCYCLE 7

WEIGHT
75.4kg

BODY FAT PERCENTAGE
7.2%

HOW TO DO THESE WORKOUTS

Do workout 42 (back and shoulders), 43 (legs) and 44 (chest and arms) in order, before advancing to the next microcycle. Never work out on more than two consecutive days.

Back and shoulders

EXERCISE	SETS	REPS	TEMPO	REST
SET 1				
1a Pull-up	3	8	4010	10sec
1b Dumbbell pull-over	3	10	3111	0sec
1c Seated cable row	3	12	3010	90sec
SET 2				
2a Reverse bench row	3	12	3011	0sec
2b Seated dumbbell shoulder press	3	10	4010	90sec
SET 3				
3a Incline reverse dumbbell flye	3	20	2010	0sec
3b Face pull	3	20	2010	90sec

1a Pull-up

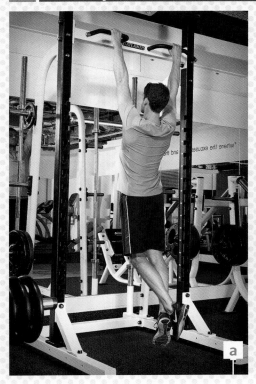 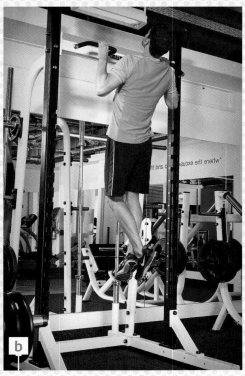

- Grab the bar with an overhand grip with your hands shoulder-width apart.
- Start from a dead hang with your arms fully extended.
- Pull yourself up by squeezing your lats together.
- Once your chin is higher than your hands pause briefly, then slowly lower yourself back to the start.

a b

1b Dumbbell pull-over

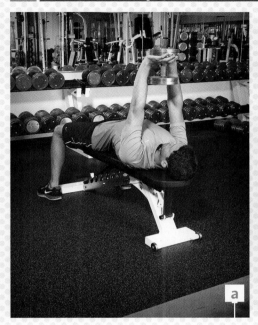

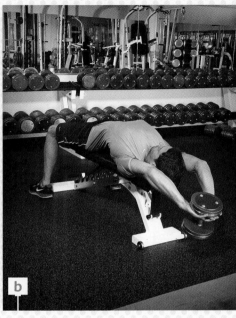

a

b

- Lie flat on a bench with your head and shoulders supported and your feet flat on the floor.
- Hold a single dumbbell over your chest with both hands and engage your core.
- Slowly lower the weight behind your head, keeping a slight bend in your elbows. Don't arch your back.
- Raise the weight back over your head to the start position.

TRAINER TIP

- The more you concentrate on using your back muscles the more successful you'll be at recruiting them.

1c Seated cable row

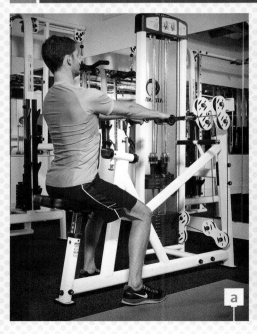

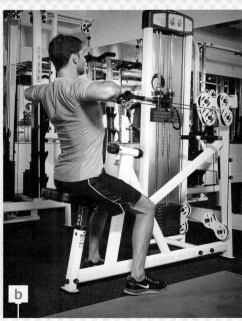

a

b

- Sit on the seat holding D-handle in each hand.
- Make sure there is tension in the cable before you begin.
- Pull the handles in to your sternum, keeping upper-body movement to a minimum, and squeeze your shoulder blades together.
- Return slowly to the start.

2a Reverse bench row

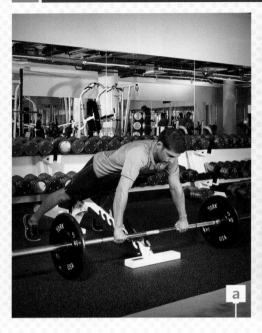
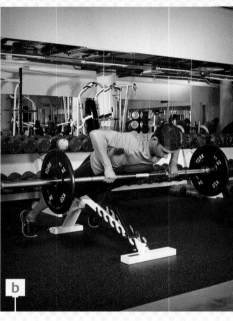

- Lie chest-first on an incline bench holding a barbell with a wide overhand grip.
- Keeping your chest on the bench, row the barbell up, leading with your elbows.
- Return to the start.

2b Seated dumbbell shoulder press

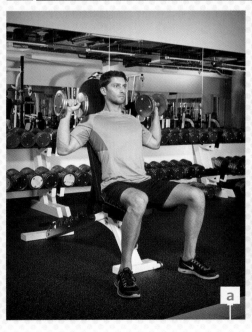
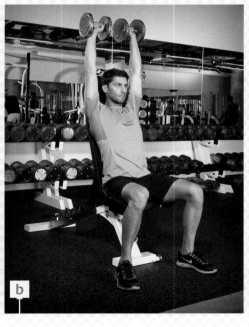

- Sit on an upright bench holding a dumbbell in each hand at shoulder height.
- Keep your feet flat on the floor, your core braced, your back against the bench and your head looking forward.
- Press the weights up powerfully until your arms are fully extended then return slowly to the start.

3a Incline reverse dumbbell flye

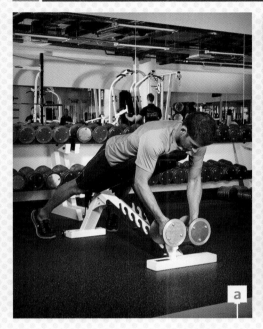
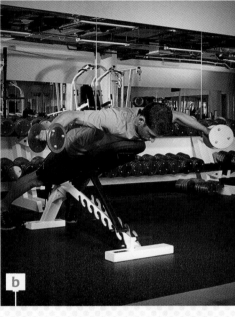

- Lie chest-forward on an incline bench holding a dumbbell in each hand.
- With a slight bend in your elbows, raise the weights out to your side until they reach shoulder height, then return to the start.

3b Face pull

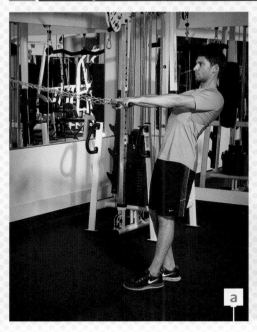
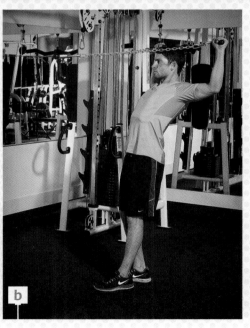

- Hold a double-rope attachment that's fixed to the high pulley on a cable machine.
- Start with your arms fully extended and your palms facing the floor.
- Pull the handles towards your head – keeping your upper arms parallel to the floor – so that the handles go to either side of your face.
- Return to the start.

Legs

EXERCISE	SETS	REPS	TEMPO	REST
SET 1				
1 Squat	5	12	4010	60sec
SET 2				
2a Walking dumbbell lunge	5	70m	X	120sec
2b Reverse sled drag	5	70m	X	180sec
SET 3				
3 Calf raise	4	15	2010	90sec

1a Squat

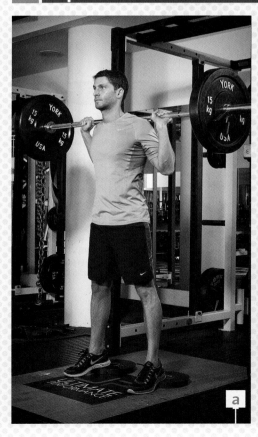
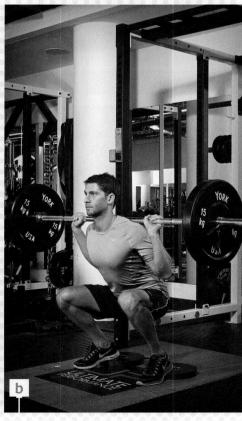

○ Rest the bar against the back of your shoulders – not on your neck – and hold it with an overhand grip slightly wider than your shoulders. Keep your elbows pointing down.

○ Your feet should be just wider than shoulder–width apart with your toes pointing outwards slightly.

○ Squat down until your thighs are at least parallel to the floor. The deeper you can squat, the better.

○ Drive back up through your heels.

2a Walking dumbbell lunge

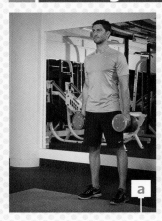
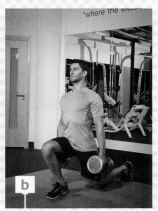

- Stand in front of a long, clear pathway holding a dumbbell in each hand.
- Keeping your core braced, take a big step forward and lunge down until both knees are bent at 90°.

- Push off from your back foot and lunge forward with that leg.
- Repeat until you have covered the stated distance.

2b Reverse sled drag

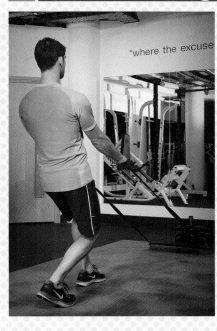

- Stand facing away from a long, clear pathway holding a sled strap in each hand.
- Keeping your core braced and your arms straight, sprint backwards as fast as you can.
- At the end, turn around and sprint back to the start.

3 Calf raise

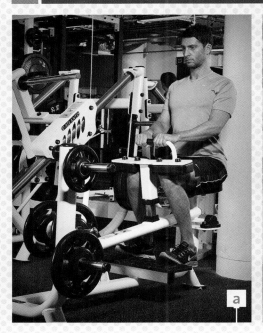
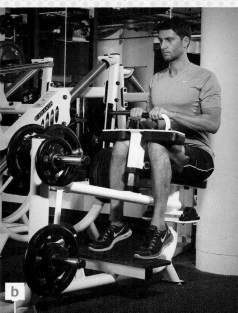

- Sit on the machine – having adjusted the weight plates or stack, depending on the equipment – with your toes on the platform.
- Release the safety catch and go up on to your tiptoes, keeping your body stable.
- Pause briefly before returning to the start, ensuring that your heel goes below the level of the platform for a full range of motion.

TRAINER TIP

- This is going to burn, but keep going through a full range of motion at the right tempo to complete the set.

Chest and arms

EXERCISE	SETS	REPS	TEMPO	REST
SET 1				
1 Incline dumbbell bench press	3	10	4010	90sec
SET 2				
2a **Incline dumbbell flye**	3	10	3110	0sec
2b **Triceps dip**	3	10	4010	90sec
SET 3				
3a **Incline dumbbell curl**	3	10	3111	0sec
3b **Decline EZ-bar triceps press**	3	12	4010	90sec
SET 4				
4a **EZ-bar preacher curl**	3	10	3010	0sec
4b **Standing overhead cable triceps extension**	3	10	3010	90sec

1 | Incline dumbbell bench press

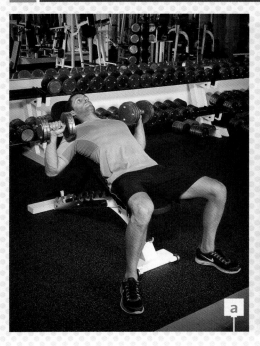
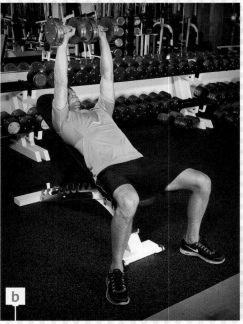

a   b

- Lie on a bench set at a 45° angle holding a dumbbell in each hand at shoulder-height.
- Keep your feet flat on the floor and your back against the bench.
- Press the weight directly above your head but don't lock out your elbows at the top.
- Slowly lower the weight back down to your chest, flaring your elbows out to the side.

TRAINER TIP

- Remember to flare your elbows out at the bottom of each rep to achieve better pectoral recruitment.

2a Incline dumbbell flye

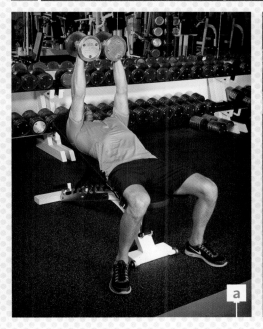
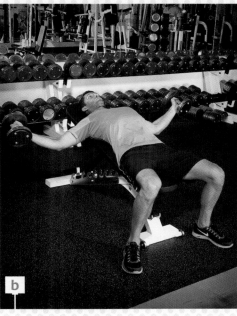

a b

- Lie on an incline bench holding a dumbbell in each hand directly above your chest with palms facing.
- Make sure your head and upper back are supported on the bench and that your feet are flat on the floor.
- Keeping a slight bend in your elbows, slowly lower the weights out to the side as far as is comfortable.
- Use your chest to reverse the movement and raise the weights back to the top.

2b Triceps dip

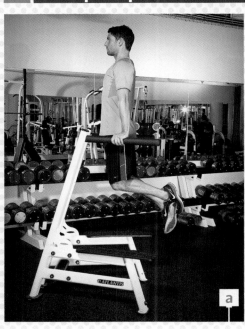
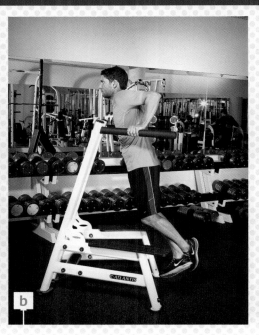

a b

- Grip parallel bars, keeping your body upright.
- With your elbows pointing straight back, lower your body as far as you can comfortably go without stressing your shoulders.
- Keep your core braced and don't swing your legs for momentum.
- Press back up powerfully but don't lock out your elbows at the top.

3a Incline dumbbell curl

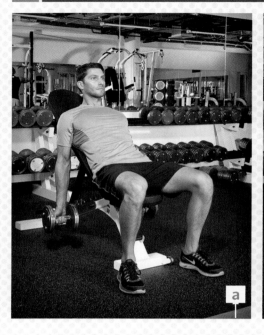
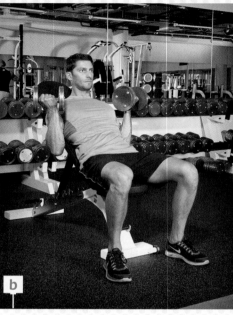

- Sit on a bench set at an incline of between 30° and 45° holding a dumbbell in each hand.
- Keeping your back flat against the bench and your elbows close to your sides, slowly curl both dumbbells up to shoulder height.
- Squeeze your biceps at the top of the move before slowly returning the start.

TRAINER TIP

- Cock your wrists back to take your forearms out of the equation. You'll lift less weight but you'll blitz your biceps.

3b Decline EZ-bar triceps press

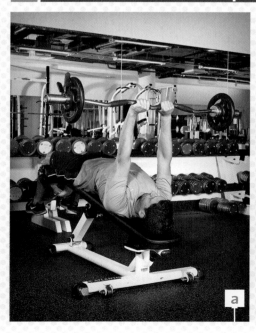
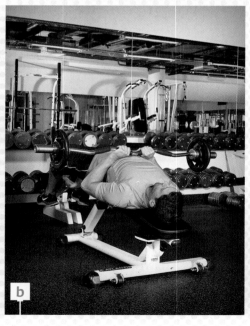

- Lie flat on a bench holding an EZ-bar with a close, overhand grip. Aim to have a fist-sized gap between your hands.
- Keep your head, shoulders and back supported by the bench with your core braced and feet flat on the floor.
- Lower the bar slowly to your chest, keeping your elbows close to your sides to keep the emphasis on your triceps.
- Push back up powerfully, but don't lock out your elbows.

TRAINER TIP

- Tuck in your elbows to put the emphasis on the triceps. As you tire, let them flare out to bring your chest into play.

4a EZ-bar preacher curl

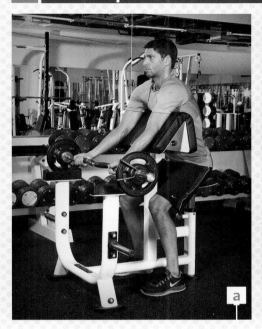
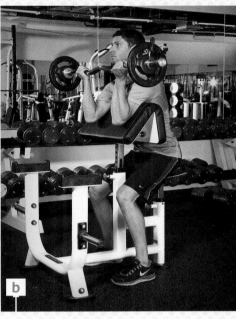

- Sit at a preacher bench holding an EZ-bar with an underhand grip.
- Keeping your elbows on the bench, curl the bar up towards your chin.
- Lower back slowly to the start.
- Avoid rocking back and forth to generate momentum, which takes the emphasis away from the biceps.

TRAINER TIP

- Squeeze your biceps at the top and flex your triceps at the bottom of each rep.

4b Standing overhead triceps extension

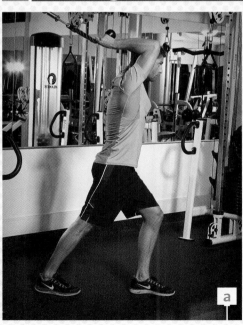
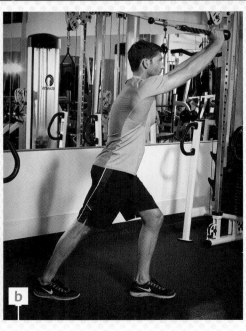

- Stand tall, holding a double-rope handle attached to the low pulley of a cable machine.
- Turn away from the machine with your hands behind your head and your elbows at either side.
- Keeping your elbows next to your head, press the handles up and forward to straighten your arms.
- Flex your triceps at the top of the move, then return to the start and flex your biceps.

WORKOUTS
45 TO 46

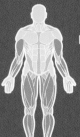

LEGS AND
ARMS
P126

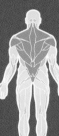

CHEST, BACK AND
SHOULDERS
P130

45 | 46

FINE-TUNING

Deplete your muscles' energy stores to make them pop

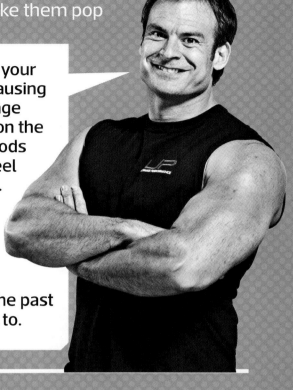

This final microcycle is designed to deplete your muscle cells of their glycogen rather than causing more muscular damage, because at this stage you're preparing your body to look its best on the big day. If you then carb-load all the fuel floods into your muscles, making them look and feel fuller and bigger – perfect for a cover shoot.

Although these two sessions are low-volume compared with the ones you've been doing, they're still tough and you may feel as if you're lifting through treacle during each set. Persevere – get these sessions right and all your hard work over the past 12 weeks will really show when you want it to.

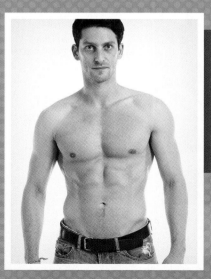

MICROCYCLE 8

WEIGHT
74.8kg

BODY FAT
PERCENTAGE
6.1%

HOW TO DO THESE WORKOUTS

Do workout 45 (legs and arms) and 46 (chest, back and shoulders) in order. Never work out on more than two consecutive days.

Legs and arms

EXERCISE	SETS	REPS	TEMPO	REST
SET 1				
1a Walking dumbbell lunge	5	40m	2010	0sec
1b Hex bar deadlift	5	20	2010	0sec
1c Lying hamstring curl	5	10	2011	0 sec
1d Sissy squat	5	15	2010	120sec
SET 2				
2a Incline dumbbell curl	4	15	2010	0sec
2b Decline EZ-bar triceps press	4	15	2010	0sec
2c Incline hammer curl	4	15	2011	0 sec
2d Decline EZ-bar triceps extension	4	15	2010	90sec

1a Walking dumbbell lunge

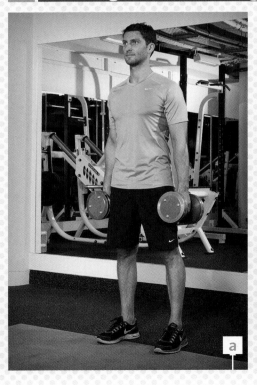
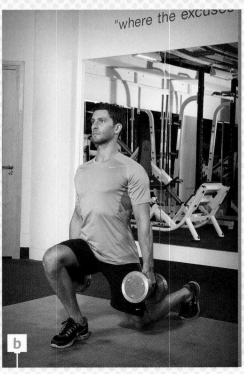

- Stand in front of a long, clear pathway holding a dumbbell in each hand.
- Keeping your core braced, take a big step forward and lunge down until both knees are bent at 90°.
- Push off from your back foot and lunge forward with that leg.
- Repeat until you have covered the stated distance.

TRAINER TIP

- A steady rhythm is key. You will want to stop, but fix your eyes on the end point and keep moving.

1b Hex bar deadlift

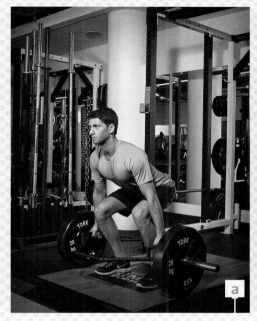

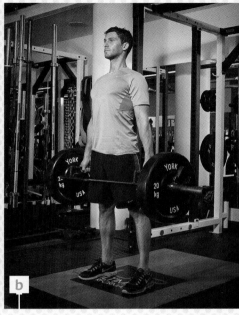

- Stand with a hex bar in front of you. Squat down, keeping your chest up, and take hold of a handle on each side.
- Use your glutes to power the initial lift, pushing down through your heels.
- As the bar passes your knees, push your hips forward, then lower the weight so that it just touches the floor before repeating.

TRAINER TIP

- If your gym doesn't have this piece of kit you can use dumbbells instead, holding one in each hand.

1c Lying hamstring curl

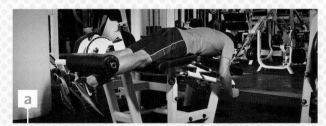

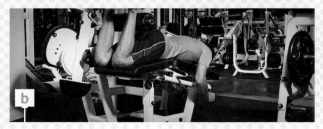

- Lie on the machine, following its instructions to position yourself correctly and safely.
- With the pad against the back of your lower calves,

- raise it up by contracting your hamstrings.
- Return slowly to the start.

1d Sissy squat

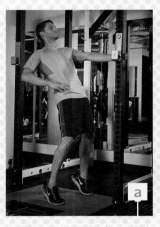

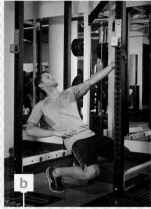

- With your feet shoulder–width apart, go up on to the balls of your feet holding a bench or other stable object for balance – but not for support.
- Squat down as deep as you can, thrusting your hips forward until you feel a good

stretch in your quads.
- Your torso will lean back and your knees will go ahead of your toes.
- Raise yourself four–fifths of the way to the start position and then squat down again.

2a Incline dumbbell curl

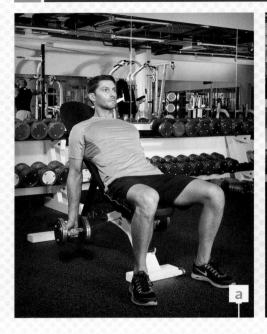
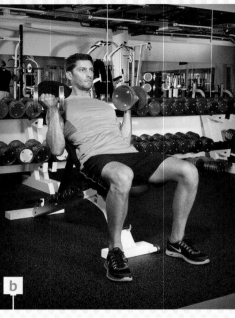

- Sit on a bench set at an incline of between 30° and 45° holding a dumbbell in each hand.
- Keeping your back flat against the bench and your elbows close to your sides, slowly curl both dumbbells up to shoulder height.
- Squeeze your biceps at the top of the move before slowly returning to the start.

2b Decline EZ-bar triceps press

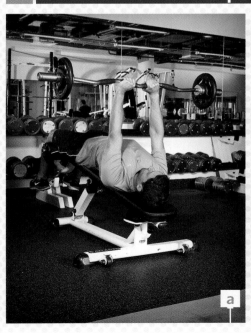
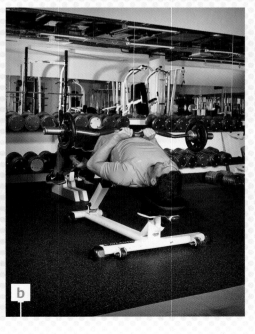

- Lie on a decline bench holding an EZ-bar above you with straight arms.
- Slowly lower the weights towards your chest, keeping your elbows close to your sides throughout.
- Press back up strongly to the start.

2c Incline hammer curl

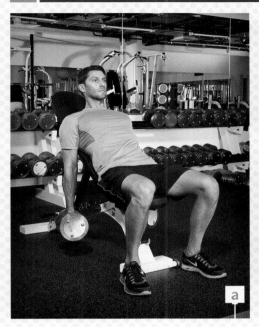
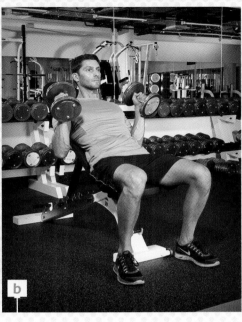

a   b

- Sit on an upright bench holding a dumbbell in each hand with your palms facing each other.
- Keeping your elbows close to your sides, slowly raise both dumbbells to shoulder height, squeezing your biceps at the top of the move.
- Slowly return the weights to the start position and repeat.

2d Decline EZ-bar triceps extension

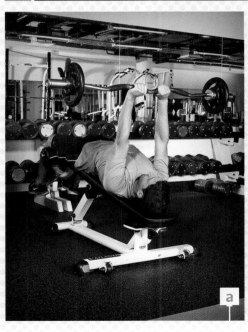
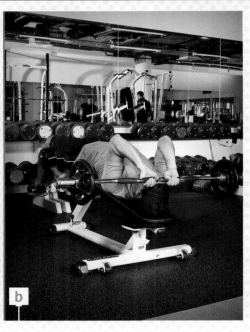

a   b

- Lie on a decline bench holding an EZ-bar above you with straight arms.
- Slowly lower the bar towards the top of your head by bending your elbows, which should point at the ceiling throughout.
- Without arching your back, slowly return the bar to the start position by straightening your arms.

Chest, back and shoulders

EXERCISE	SETS	REPS	TEMPO	REST
SET 1				
1a Chin-up	3	12	2010	0sec
1b Triceps dip	3	15	2010	75sec
SET 2				
2a Reverse bench row	3	12	2010	0sec
2b Incline dumbbell bench press	3	12	2010	75sec
SET 3				
3a Seated cable row	3	15	3010	0sec
3b Dumbbell bench press	3	15	3010	75sec
SET 4				
4a Face pull	3	15	2011	0sec
4b Cable crossover	3	25	3011	60sec

1a Chin-up

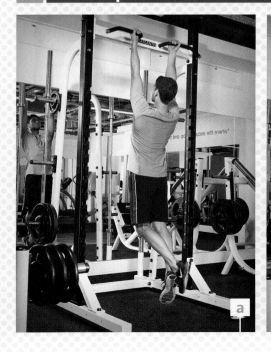
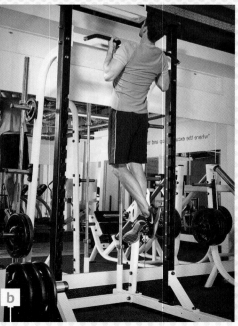

- Grab the bar with an underhand grip with your hands shoulder-width apart.
- Start from a dead hang with your arms fully extended.
- Pull yourself up by squeezing your lats together.
- Once your chin is higher than your hands, lower yourself back to the start.

TRAINER TIP

- Always go to full extension at the bottom of each rep to work your muscles through their full range of motion.

1b | Triceps dip

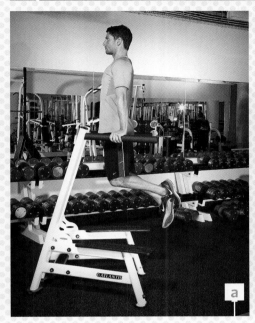

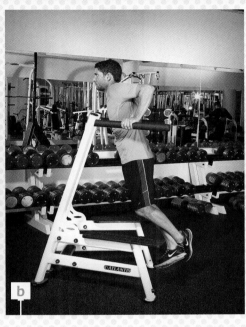

- Grip parallel bars, keeping your body upright.
- With your elbows pointing straight back, lower your body as far as you can comfortably go without stressing your shoulders.
- Keep your core braced and don't swing your legs for momentum.
- Press back up powerfully but don't lock out your elbows at the top.

2a | Reverse bench row

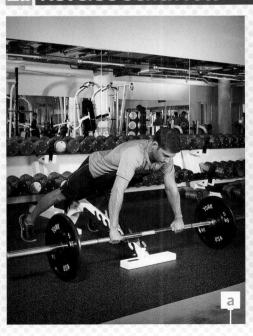

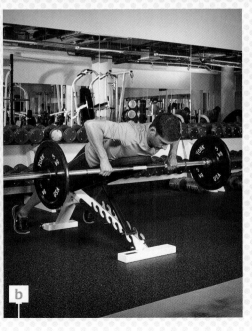

- Lie chest-first on an incline bench holding a barbell with a wide overhand grip.
- Keeping your chest on the bench, row the barbell up, leading with your elbows.
- Return to the start.

2b Incline dumbbell bench press

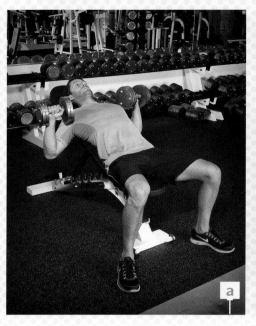
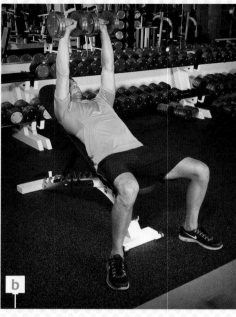

- Lie on a bench set at a 45° angle holding a dumbbell in each hand at shoulder-height.
- Keep your feet flat on the floor and your back against the bench.
- Press the weight directly above your head but don't lock out your elbows at the top. Return to the start.

3a Seated cable row

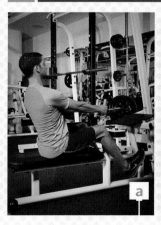
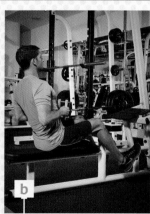

3b Dumbbell bench press

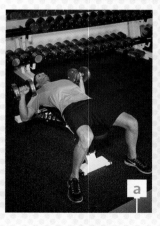
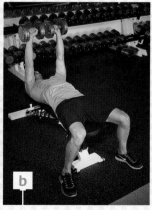

- Sit on the bench with a slight bend in your knees holding a double-D handle – attached to the lower pulley of a cable machine – with a neutral grip.
- Ensure that there is tension in the cable before you begin.
- Pull the handle in to your sternum, keeping upper-body movement to a minimum, and squeeze your shoulder blades together.
- Return slowly to the start.

- Lie on a flat bench holding a dumbbell in each hand at shoulder height.
- Keep your feet flat on the floor and your back against the bench.
- Press the weight directly above your head but don't lock out your elbows at the top. Return to the start.

4a Face pull

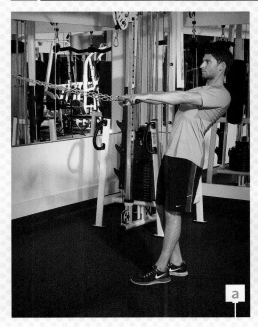 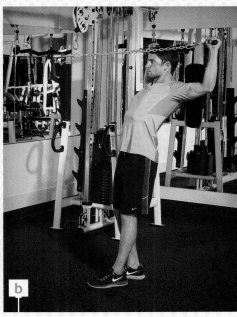

a
b

- Hold a double-rope attachment that's fixed to the high pulley on a cable machine.
- Start with your arms fully extended and your palms facing the floor.
- Pull the handles towards your head – keeping your upper arms parallel to the floor – so that the handles go to either side of your face.
- Return to the start.

4b Cable crossover

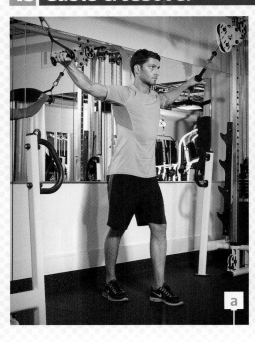 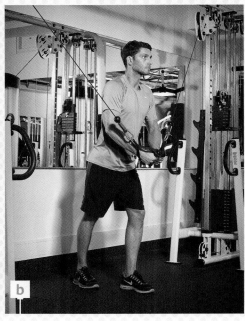

a
b

- Stand in the middle of a cable machine with a split stance holding a D-handle attachment in each hand, with the cable set above shoulder height.
- Keeping a natural arch in your back, your core braced and upper body still, bring your hands down in an arc to meet in front of your chest.
- Pause briefly and squeeze your chest muscles before returning slowly to the start, keeping the weight under full control.

TRAINER TIP

- To get more out of each rep, think about your chest muscles squeezing to bring the handles together.

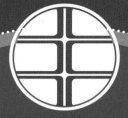

ABS AND FAT LOSS

Carve a rock-hard six-pack and blast away the last traces of fat to complete your transformation

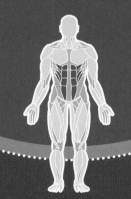

GET A SIX-PACK

Use this chapter to develop rock-hard abs

If you've followed this programme to the letter then you've strongly stacked the odds of possessing a genuinely impressive six-pack in your favour. However, if you're like Joe, genetics may be holding you back a touch and preventing your now leaner stomach from exhibiting hard abs. Don't worry, that's easy to fix. This chapter contains all the advice you need to work your abs and build greater muscle mass and thickness, which will really make them stand out. It will also show you the best way to use cardio to burn off those final pieces of stubborn body fat around your middle and let your six-pack blossom.

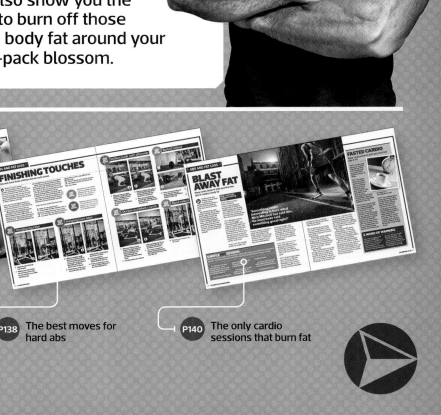

P136 The science behind getting a six-pack

P138 The best moves for hard abs

P140 The only cardio sessions that burn fat

SIX-PACK SCIENCE

Struggling to reveal your abs despite endless crunches? It's probably because you're doing the wrong exercise. Here's everything you need to know about getting the perfect six-pack

What is a six-pack?

A Anatomically speaking, the six-pack is the rectus abdominus, a paired muscle that runs vertically on each side of the front of the abdomen, separated down the middle by a band of connective tissue called the linea alba, or white line. It's this line and those that run horizontally across this muscle group that create the six distinct parts of a six-pack.

What does this muscle do?

A It's an important postural muscle responsible for flexing your spine forwards. It also assists with breathing, stabilises the torso during exercise and protects your internal organs from impact.

Why can't I see mine?

A Everyone has a six-pack but most people can't see

theirs for one simple reason: it's hidden under a layer of fat. Men are predisposed to storing body fat around the stomach, whereas women keep theirs on their hips and bottom. If you have excess body fat, it's going to prevent your abs from being on full display.

What's the best way to lose belly fat?

A For years people have believed – wrongly – that lots of cardio training in the 'fat-burning zone' was the only way to shift body fat (see box, below). In fact, the best way to effectively burn away excess fat is by doing weight training and high-intensity cardio, such as sprints.

These approaches increase your heart rate and your metabolism (the rate at which your body burns calories), so your fat stores have to be used as fuel. You also need to follow a high-protein diet and control your intake of carbohydrates,

which flood your body with energy that not only prevents you from burning fat but also increases fat stores if you don't use up all that energy.

Which exercises are more effective at building hard abs?

A Heavy compound lifts, such as squats, deadlifts and overhead presses, work the entire abdominal region far harder than sit-ups or crunches. That's because the six-pack muscles are responsible for stabilising your torso and must therefore work hard to keep your upper body in a stable, secure position whenever you lift heavy weights. However, exercises that directly target the abs should also be included in any training programme to work the muscles as hard as possible and promote maximum growth.

What moves are best for directly targeting the abs?

A Not sit-ups, despite the widespread view that they are. They allow the hip flexor muscles to dominate the move, not the abs, so they'll never build a six-pack regardless of the hours you dedicate to them. Planks, however, are great for building strength in the deep-lying stability muscles of the core. Weighted crunches hit the top of the abs, and knee and leg raises target the lower abs, while barbell

rollouts work everything. All these moves are detailed on the following pages.

Are low-rep or high-rep sets of abs moves the most effective?

A Every muscle group is predominately made of either fast-twitch or slow-twitch muscle fibres. The abs are mainly fast-twitch, which means they typically respond better to heavy-weight, low-rep sets. That said, you should still do a combination of low-rep and high-rep abs moves to tax the muscle fibres as much as possible and ensure greater returns.

Is it also important to work the muscles in my lower back?

A Your lower back muscles are an important but often overlooked part of your core. They play a huge role in stabilising your torso and assisting in the transfer of power between your upper and lower body.

Failing to dedicate the same amount of training time to your lower back as you do to your abs will result in an unbalanced core that will at best prevent your abs from developing to their full potential and at worst result in injury. This workout includes plenty of lower-back moves, which is why it also provides a huge amount of direct abs work to allow your six-pack to blossom.

THE FAT-BURNING ZONE MYTH

If long, slow, steady-state cardio exercise was the best way to burn fat, then everyone who ran the London Marathon would cross the finish line with abs of steel. Although this type of training does burn calories, it doesn't actually produce optimum fat loss. That's because too much steady-state exercise can actually decrease the

levels of muscle-building, fat-burning testosterone and growth hormone, and increase levels of the stress hormone cortisol.

High cortisol levels prompt your body to store energy as abdominal fat and break down muscle for energy too. So keep cardio sessions short and intense and get ripped faster.

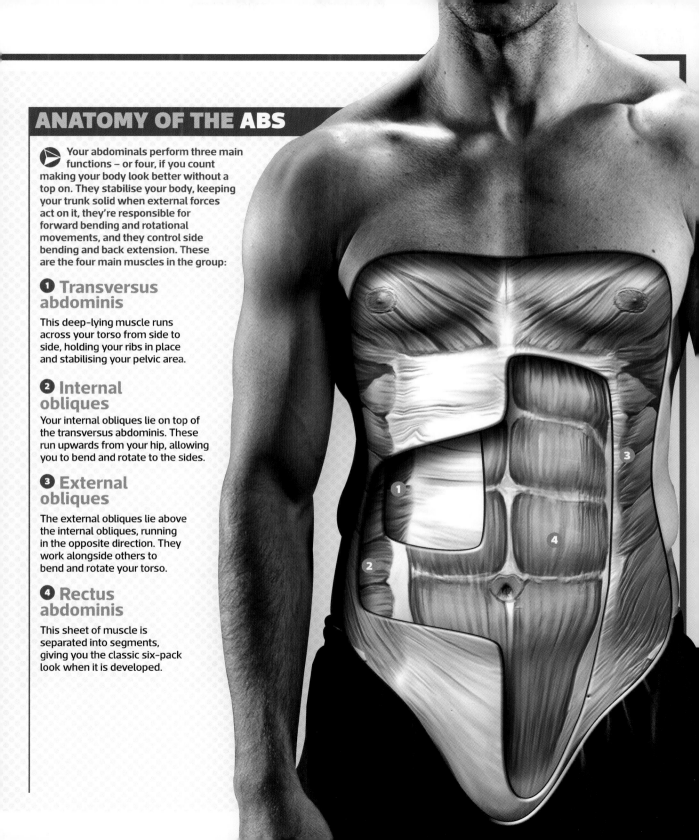

ANATOMY OF THE ABS

Your abdominals perform three main functions – or four, if you count making your body look better without a top on. They stabilise your body, keeping your trunk solid when external forces act on it, they're responsible for forward bending and rotational movements, and they control side bending and back extension. These are the four main muscles in the group:

❶ Transversus abdominis

This deep-lying muscle runs across your torso from side to side, holding your ribs in place and stabilising your pelvic area.

❷ Internal obliques

Your internal obliques lie on top of the transversus abdominis. These run upwards from your hip, allowing you to bend and rotate to the sides.

❸ External obliques

The external obliques lie above the internal obliques, running in the opposite direction. They work alongside others to bend and rotate your torso.

❹ Rectus abdominis

This sheet of muscle is separated into segments, giving you the classic six-pack look when it is developed.

TARGET YOUR ABS

Get rock-hard abs by adding extra six-pack moves to your workout

While it's true that heavy compound lifts, such as squats, deadlifts and shoulder presses, will work your abs, to build a rock-hard six-pack you need to target your abs directly with exercises that place them under a lot of stress so they have the stimulus to grow to their maximum potential.

Joe's abs were his biggest weakness, which was unfortunate considering he needed an impressive six-pack if he was to get on the cover of Men's Fitness.

His genetics were to blame. Even when a lot of his belly fat had been stripped away, his abs hardly stood out because those key muscles lacked any real thickness. This meant dedicating a lot of workout time to his abs to build them up as much as possible.

Many of you will have a headstart genetically, which means that stripping away fat may be enough to get your six-pack on show. If so, the abs moves included in the 12-week programme will be enough to bring them out in great detail. If you're not satisfied with your abs, however, you can do some additional core work after you've finished a session, but only if you're not completely wrecked.

If you do, here are the three key rules:

1 Never do abs exercises on consecutive sessions. Always leave at least one workout between core moves.

2 Pick one high-rep move and one low-rep move. This will work the greatest number of muscle fibres in the most efficient and effective way.

3 Do four sets of 6-12 reps for the low-rep moves and 20-30 reps for the high-rep moves.

HIGH REP MOVE These moves place less resistance on your abs so they can be performed in high-rep sets to work the muscles thoroughly.

LOW REP MOVE These moves place greater resistance on your abs so each rep is far harder.

HIGH REP MOVE — Hanging leg raise

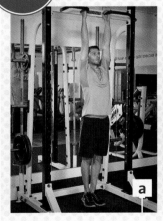
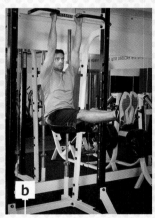

- **a** Hang from a bar with your body straight.
- **b** Keeping your legs straight, use your lower abs to raise them until they are parallel to the ground.

HIGH REP MOVE — Hanging knee raise

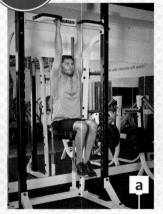
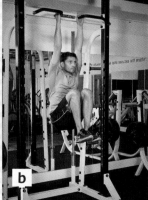

- **a** Hang from a bar with your torso straight and your knees bent to 90° with your thighs parallel to the ground.
- **b** Bring your knees up towards your chest and lower them to the start position.

Decline plank with touch

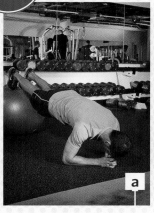
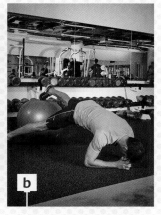

a b

- With your feet on a platform or ball, hold your body in a straight line with your elbows under your shoulders and your head looking down.

- Without letting your hips sag, lift one foot up and to the side, then lower it to the floor. Touch the ground and return to the start position. Repeat with your other leg.

Barbell rollout

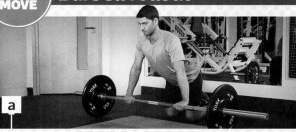

a

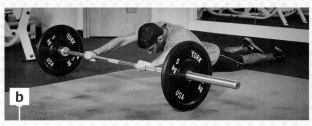

b

- Get on your knees with your arms straight and your hands holding a barbell with a shoulder-width grip.

- Slowly roll the barbell forward keeping your core braced.

- Once your torso is parallel to the floor, contract your abs to pull the bar back to the start.

Decline dumbbell crunch

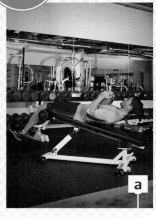
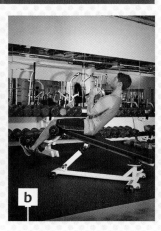

a b

- Lie on a decline bench holding a dumbbell in both hands across your chest.

- Slowly crunch up your torso then lower under control back to the start position, maintaining tension on your abs throughout the move.

Band rollout

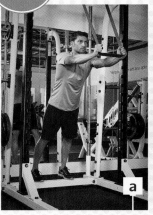
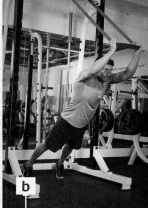

a b

- Attach a resistance band over pull-up handles and hold it with both hands. Stand so you're leaning forward slightly with tension on your abs.

- Keeping your body straight, lean forwards as far as you can go, then contract your abs to return to the start position.

BLAST AWAY FAT

Discover the best ways to shift those final few bits of stubborn body fat

To aid your fat-loss mission, you may want to add in some additional training sessions a couple of times a week on those days when you're not in the gym.

'Joe started doing some outdoor training once or twice a week about six weeks into the challenge to force his body to keep burning fat while maintaining muscle mass,' explains Nick. 'But it's no good just hitting the road for a two-hour run: the type of training you do is critically important.' Here's what you need to do and why.

High-intensity interval training, or HIIT

WHAT? HIIT is a method of intense cardiovascular training that's proven to burn body fat. Similar to weight training, it elevates your metabolism for up to 24 hours after the session so you continue to get leaner long after you have finished.

WHY? HIIT works because of a process called excess post-exercise oxygen consumption (EPOC). It creates an oxygen debt and a build-up of lactic acid in your muscles, both of which must be eradicated once you've finished exercise. As your body restores this imbalance it increases your metabolism, so you burn more calories even at rest.

WHAT ELSE? The benefits of HIIT over steady-state forms of cardiovascular exercise are numerous: it improves cardiovascular fitness and health to a far greater extent; it doesn't take as long, so doesn't get boring or repetitive; it can have profoundly positive hormonal benefits, such as raising growth hormone levels and improving insulin sensitivity; and, done correctly, it also places a nice stimulus on your muscles and therefore helps to improve your overall body composition.

STILL NEED CONVINCING? Think of the difference in physiques between a 100m sprinter and a marathon runner. The former does HIIT, the latter does long, steady-state cardio.

HOW? Unlike weight-training, when there's right way and a wrong way to train depending on your goals, if you're using HIIT as a tool to improve your body composition you'll get

> 'Pick an exercise you enjoy. If you love running but hate the rowing machine, you're more likely to stick to it if you run instead of row'

SAMPLE HIIT SESSION

Pick an exercise you like – park running, cycling, swimming or any other form of physical activity – and follow these workout instructions for an effective fat-burning session

▶ Start with 2-5 minutes at an easy, moderate pace – hard enough so you can hold a conversation if you had to.

▶ Next do 10 x 20 seconds at all-out effort alternated with 40 seconds at a slow and comfortable pace.

▶ Then 5-10 minutes of steady-state at a moderate to challenging (slightly out of breath) intensity.

▶ Next, 4 x 45 seconds' all-out effort alternated with 60 seconds at comfortable pace.

▶ Finish with 5 minutes at the same pace as your first 5 minutes.

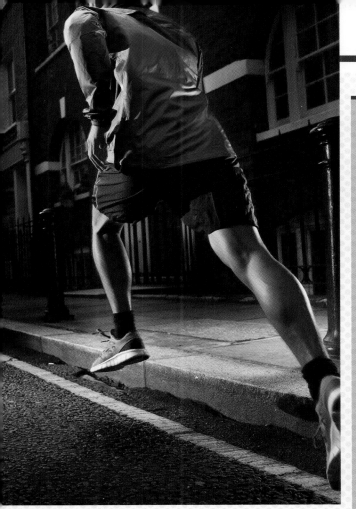

FASTED WALKING

This controversial method can have great results

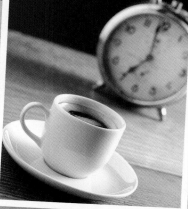

WHAT? Gentle cardio training on an empty stomach first thing in the morning can be a great way to chip away at your fat stores.

WHY? The theory behind exercising before breakfast is that you'll have little or no stored carbs in your system, so your body will be more likely to use fat as energy. Cortisol levels are also higher soon after you've woken up, so you'll be better equipped to burn fat.

WHAT ELSE? Fasted walking is a controversial topic and not a training method for everyone. If you're naturally skinny and stressed, it's too demanding on your system to exercise in a fasted state as cortisol levels can be raised too high and eat away all your hard-earned muscle. Joe is naturally skinny and prone to stress but we needed to do this because we were on a tight time frame.

HOW? When you wake up have a strong cup of black coffee to help raise your cortisol levels and provide a hit of caffeine, both of which will help to mobilise fat stores for energy. Also take about 20g of BCAAs to prevent muscle mass loss without raising insulin levels, which would be counterproductive.

The next bit is simple: go for a power walk for between 20 and 45 minutes. It's that simple.

A WORD OF WARNING

If you're struggling with energy and feel tired, fatigued or miserable, don't do this fasted session. It's more important that you have enough energy to go hard during your weight training. Fasted walking is very much the icing on the cake and should be the first thing you drop if you begin to feel you're suffering from the symptoms of overtraining.

---

far more out of it by freestyling a little bit. Just make sure you follow these key principles:

▶ Pick an exercise you enjoy. If you love running but hate the rowing machine, you're more likely to stick to it if you run instead of row.

▶ Each session can last anything from ten to 40 minutes. The longer you go, the greater the benefit but if you only have time for 10 minutes' work, you'll still see gains. Quality beats quantity.

▶ After a quick warm-up, go fast then slow, then repeat. That's all a HIIT session needs to be. It can be 30 seconds' all-out effort, followed by 45 seconds' easy, or it can be 15 seconds and 15 seconds, or 35 seconds and 60 seconds. Mix it up as much as possible because this keeps your body guessing and prevents it slipping into a 'fuel-efficiency' mode, which is what happens during steady-state cardio.

▶ Never do HIIT before weight training. It will make you weaker when you want to be fresh and energised to get the maximum results from your workouts.

▶ Don't do HIIT with too many carbs in your system. If you do, the carbs will get burned as fuel when you want to be targeting your fat stores. Carbs also raise your body's insulin levels when in fact you want these sessions to lower your insulin levels for an optimal fat-burning response.

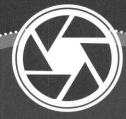

FINISHING TOUCHES

Now you've put in the hours at the gym, it's time for those final few tweaks before your transformation is complete

ALMOST THERE...

Discover how to show off your body at its best

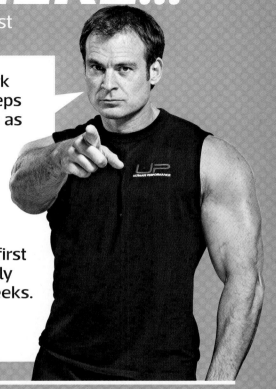

After 12 weeks, Joe had done all the hard work in the gym but there were still a few small steps he had to take in order to look as big and lean as possible ahead of the *Men's Fitness* cover shoot. And after 46 tough workouts and three months of sticking to a very specific diet, you're almost there too. These final little tips and tricks are there to ensure you look your absolute best when you want to, whether that's for your own photoshoot, the first day of your beach holiday or just to see exactly how much you really can change in just 12 weeks. Think of this chapter as the icing on the cake – not that you're allowed any cake, of course.

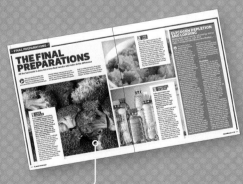

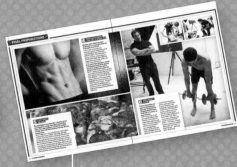

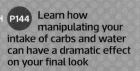

P144 Learn how manipulating your intake of carbs and water can have a dramatic effect on your final look

P146 With just days to go until the end of the programme, it's time for some last-minute tricks to make you look your best

THE FINAL COUNTDOWN

The realisation of all your hard work is just a few simple steps away

You may be finished in the gym but that doesn't mean your challenge is over just yet. In fact, there are several last-minute things you can do to make your new physique look even better, and the best bit is that they're all easy to do. Follow the steps Joe took in the final few days before his cover model shoot to add the finishing touches and show off your bigger, stronger and leaner body.

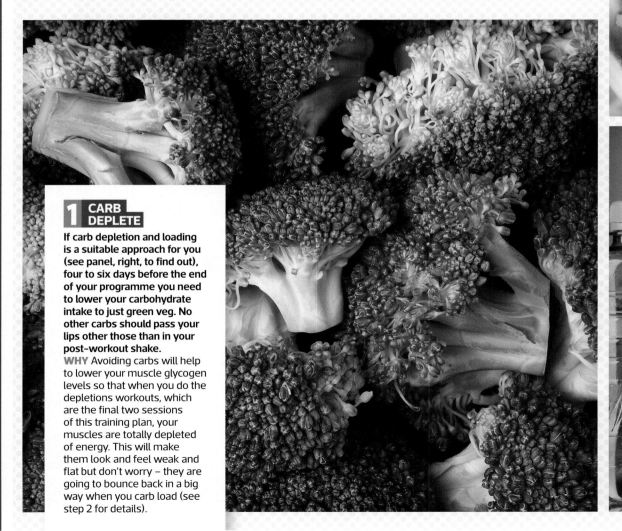

1 CARB DEPLETE

If carb depletion and loading is a suitable approach for you (see panel, right, to find out), four to six days before the end of your programme you need to lower your carbohydrate intake to just green veg. No other carbs should pass your lips other those than in your post-workout shake.

WHY Avoiding carbs will help to lower your muscle glycogen levels so that when you do the depletions workouts, which are the final two sessions of this training plan, your muscles are totally depleted of energy. This will make them look and feel weak and flat but don't worry – they are going to bounce back in a big way when you carb load (see step 2 for details).

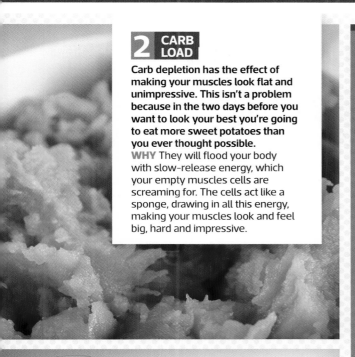

2 | CARB LOAD

Carb depletion has the effect of making your muscles look flat and unimpressive. This isn't a problem because in the two days before you want to look your best you're going to eat more sweet potatoes than you ever thought possible.

WHY They will flood your body with slow-release energy, which your empty muscles cells are screaming for. The cells act like a sponge, drawing in all this energy, making your muscles look and feel big, hard and impressive.

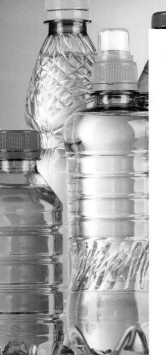

3 | DRINK LOTS OF WATER

In the week before the end of the programme, you need to increase the amount of water you drink every day to around six litres – more, if possible. A warning: you'll be going for a pee fairly often.

WHY You need to get your body used to processing vast amounts of water because the day before you take your final photos you will stop drinking. Joe stopped at 6pm the night before his cover shoot. By this time, his body was so used to excreting all the water he was drinking that it continued to do so even after he stopped. It drew all the excess water out of his skin, making him look even bigger and leaner.

DEPLETE AND LOAD

Manipulate your muscle cell energy stores to look even better, says Nick

Glycogen is a molecule made up of one part carbohydrate to four parts water, so the right type of loading can really swell your muscles. The theory behind deliberately draining your muscle cells of glycogen is that when you then load up on carbs your cells super-compensate by sucking in as much glycogen as possible, making your muscles look bigger and more defined.

However, this isn't a one-size-fits-all strategy. If five to ten days from the end of the programme you already look fantastic, there's a strong argument for not making any final alterations. I'd estimate that at least half of you won't need to go through this process.

If you don't want or need to deplete and load, stick to your normal diet. However, if you do want to do it, have a trial run two weeks before the end of the programme to see how you look and feel. You can then tweak the process to suit you.

Rules of depletion

Before you start carb depletion, there are a few simple ground rules you should follow.

The length of your carb depletion should be based on how much muscle you have: if you weigh under 75kg, deplete for 24–48 hours; 75-100kg for 24–72 hours; over 100kg for 48-72 hours. Too long a depletion can be counterproductive.

Carb depletion should be based around how you've been dieting. If you've had zero carbs you can deplete at this level, but if you've been averaging 300g dropping to zero would be too much. In such a case, take in 25% of your regular carb intake on depletion days. If you've been carb cycling, do 25% of a normal 'medium-carb' day. Still eat a decent amount of protein (2g per kilo of bodyweight) and have at least two servings of red meat.

Time to load

When it comes to carb loading, you should do it for the same amount of time as you depleted.

My basic formula for carb loading is to take your lean bodyweight in kilos and multiply it by four to get your optimal carb-loading dosage. Joe weighed 75kg, so he had 300g of carbs on loading days.

In your loading phase, protein intake should be 0.5g per kilo of bodyweight. Keep fat intake low, so avoid red meat and eggs, and stick to turkey and white fish.

Carb choices

Carb loading isn't an excuse to eat like a pig. Stick with the carbs you've been eating already. As oatmeal left Joe feeling slightly bloated, he consumed his 300g of carbs each day in the form of sweet potatoes.

On the final day (see step 5), stop counting carbs and calories altogether. Pigging out on junk food is going to make you look awesome.

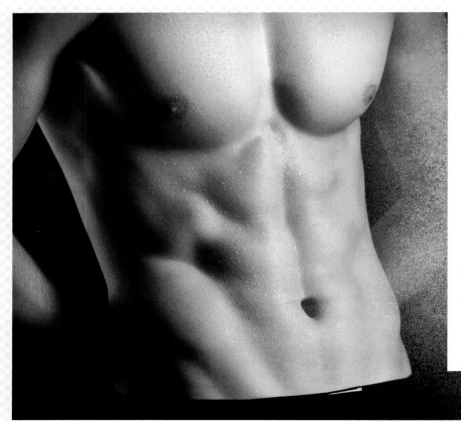

4 TRIM YOUR CHEST AND GET A TAN

Whether your chest has a few stray hairs or is covered in thick fur, it all needs to come off. And if you don't have the time, money or inclination to jet off to warmer climes for a week, you'll need to get a spray tan too.

WHY? Hair covers your muscles and can make them look average rather than hard with defined edges. The best way to get rid of hair is to use clippers to trim it right down without irritating your skin, which can occur if you wet shave.

When it comes to the skin itself, 'darker, tanned skin absorbs more light and makes the muscles look harder and more defined', says Mitchell. 'You'll look 10-20% better with a tan because it will highlight your new muscles and make you look leaner.' If you are serious about getting a good tan, book an appointment at a salon instead of nicking your girlfriend's leftovers.

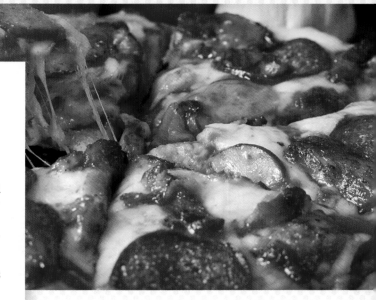

5 LAST-NIGHT RELOAD

The night before his shoot, Joe received a phone call from Nick telling him to order in a large meat pizza and to eat four slices. The only condition was that he couldn't actually eat them until the following morning. At 6am, to be precise.

WHY? Joe's shoot began at 11am, so Nick wanted him to eat a high-carb, high-fat, high-sodium meal first thing in the morning to accelerate the process of driving fluid into his muscle cells. Then, at 9am, Nick told Joe to visit any fast-food place and get two breakfast burgers, ideally with either bacon or sausage. It's these higher fat, high-salt foods that he'd been avoiding like the plague for the last 12 weeks that would actually help get him looking his best when the camera started snapping.

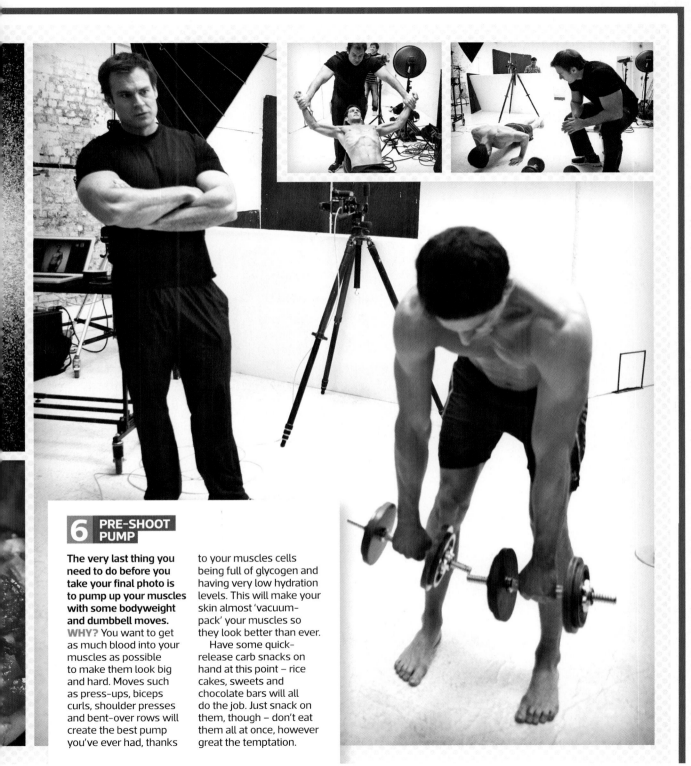

6 PRE-SHOOT PUMP

The very last thing you need to do before you take your final photo is to pump up your muscles with some bodyweight and dumbbell moves.
WHY? You want to get as much blood into your muscles as possible to make them look big and hard. Moves such as press-ups, biceps curls, shoulder presses and bent-over rows will create the best pump you've ever had, thanks to your muscles cells being full of glycogen and having very low hydration levels. This will make your skin almost 'vacuum-pack' your muscles so they look better than ever.

Have some quick-release carb snacks on hand at this point – rice cakes, sweets and chocolate bars will all do the job. Just snack on them, though – don't eat them all at once, however great the temptation.

COMPLETE GUIDE TO NUTRITION

In this chapter you'll discover everything you need to know about what you should be eating – and when – to make sure you hit your targets

FOOD FOR A BIGGER, LEANER BODY

What you eat is as important as how you train

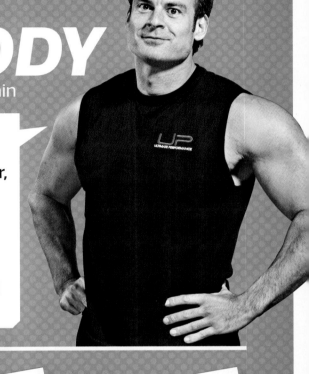

You can't out-train a bad diet. It may be an old fitness cliché but it stands true. Even if you follow every single workout to the letter, you won't end up with a cover model body at the end of the 12 weeks if you don't do the same with your diet. This chapter is all about what you need to eat and – crucially – when, because the timing of your meals is important to ensure you build muscle and burn fat when your body is primed to do so.

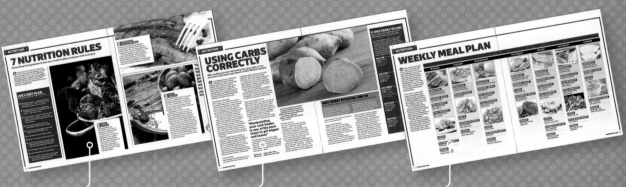

P150 Follow Nick's seven simple nutrition rules to make sure you maximise your muscle-building potential in the gym

P154 Discover the role carbs have to play in your eating plan over the next 12 weeks, including the concept of carb cycling

P156 Now you know the rules, find out how to put them into action with a typical seven-day meal plan as followed by Joe Warner

7 NUTRITION RULES

Follow these food guidelines to fuel your muscle-building challenge while burning fat

What you eat is every bit as important to the success of this challenge as what you do in the gym. Here are the seven rules you'll need to live by over the next 12 weeks. The good news is it's much more simple than you'd think. But to reach your target you'll need to be as organised in the kitchen as you are in the weights room.

JOE'S DIET PLAN
Nick gave Joe a list of maxims to stick to

- Breakfast is meat – preferably red and preferably beef – with a handful of nuts (remember, peanuts are not nuts).

- Eat green and cruciferous vegetables – preferably broccoli, cauliflower, spinach or kale – with every meal.

- All fats should come from red meat and oily fish only. In addition, you can also eat three to six whole eggs, three to four times a week.

- Aim to eat 4g protein per kilo of bodyweight, spread over six meals.

- You can eat two servings of red meat a day but avoid the fattier cuts.

- Limit pork to two servings a week.

- Drink 2.5-4 litres of water every day.

- Portion size is simple: a normal-size plate must be filled half with greens and half with protein. Nothing else.

- One whey protein shake a day, no more.

- Cook with butter, not vegetable oil.

- Avoid alcohol. One medium-size glass of red wine is allowed on a Saturday night. If you think it's worth it.

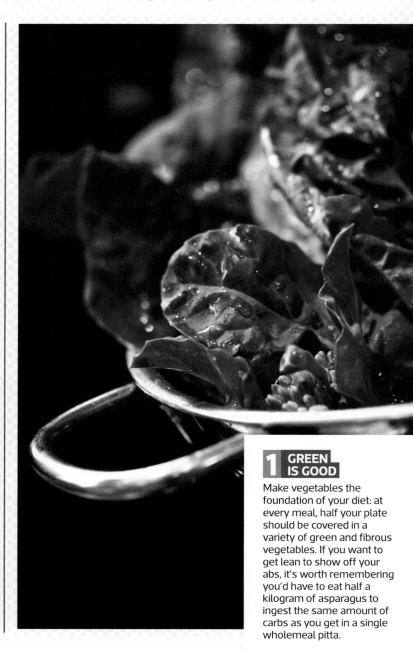

1 GREEN IS GOOD

Make vegetables the foundation of your diet: at every meal, half your plate should be covered in a variety of green and fibrous vegetables. If you want to get lean to show off your abs, it's worth remembering you'd have to eat half a kilogram of asparagus to ingest the same amount of carbs as you get in a single wholemeal pitta.

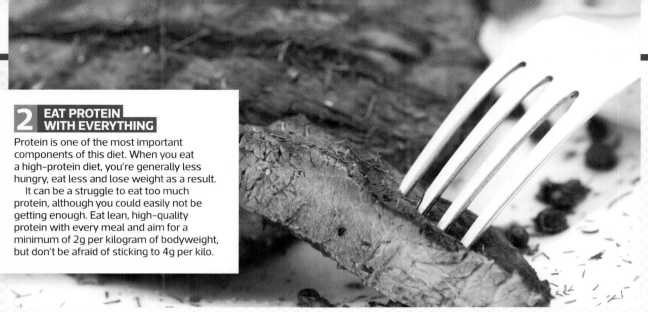

2 EAT PROTEIN WITH EVERYTHING

Protein is one of the most important components of this diet. When you eat a high-protein diet, you're generally less hungry, eat less and lose weight as a result.

It can be a struggle to eat too much protein, although you could easily not be getting enough. Eat lean, high-quality protein with every meal and aim for a minimum of 2g per kilogram of bodyweight, but don't be afraid of sticking to 4g per kilo.

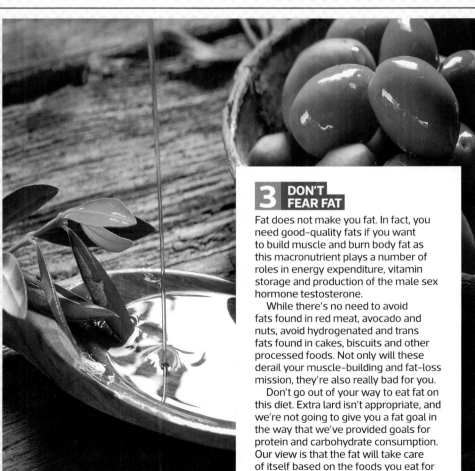

3 DON'T FEAR FAT

Fat does not make you fat. In fact, you need good-quality fats if you want to build muscle and burn body fat as this macronutrient plays a number of roles in energy expenditure, vitamin storage and production of the male sex hormone testosterone.

While there's no need to avoid fats found in red meat, avocado and nuts, avoid hydrogenated and trans fats found in cakes, biscuits and other processed foods. Not only will these derail your muscle-building and fat-loss mission, they're also really bad for you.

Don't go out of your way to eat fat on this diet. Extra lard isn't appropriate, and we're not going to give you a fat goal in the way that we've provided goals for protein and carbohydrate consumption. Our view is that the fat will take care of itself based on the foods you eat for your protein intake.

'Fat does not make you fat. In fact, you need to good-quality fats if you want to build muscle and burn body fat'

4 MACRONUTRIENTS ARE MORE IMPORTANT THAN CALORIES

Here's a quick lesson in logic if you're still locked into the old-school 'calories in, calories out' rule for fat loss. What's going to make you fatter: 2,000 calories from ice cream or 2,000 calories from white fish and veg? You know the answer to this already, so you should accept that the intake of the correct macronutrients is ultimately more significant than mere calorie counting.

That said, calories – or more significantly, portion control – are still a key consideration when wanting to lose fat. Think of the impact on body composition of 2,000 calories from white fish and veg to that of 5,000 calories from the same foods. Remember, the aim is to get to single-digit body-fat levels, so you want to hit the right macronutrient numbers to build muscle without eating any unnecessary calories.

5 START AS YOU MEAN TO GO ON

Think of breakfast like any other meal: you need a blend of protein, fats and veg. At first it may be strange to eat steak with broccoli first thing, but eating the right foods for breakfast will set you up for the rest of the day, get your metabolism firing and start the supply of quality nutrients to your muscles.

6 FREE-RANGE IS KEY

Free-range animals have more varied diets and get a lot more exercise, allowing the development of more muscle, which in turn tends to contain more zinc, vitamins B, A and K, amino acids, iron, selenium, phosphorus and zinc. Also, farm-raised salmon has also been found to contain up to eight times the level of carcinogens as its wild brethren, thanks to cramped conditions and poor-quality feed, while grass-fed beef tends to have much higher levels of conjugated linoleic acid and omega 3s than the kind fed on grain.

Eating free-range feels less like a frivolous luxury if you think of it this way: it's so nutritionally dissimilar to cage-reared that it's basically different food.

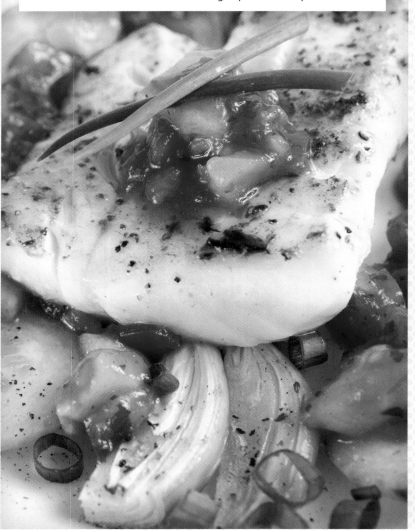

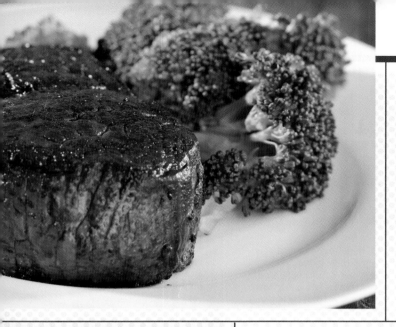

'What's going to make you fatter: 2,000 calories from ice cream or 2,000 calories from white fish and veg? You know the answer to this already'

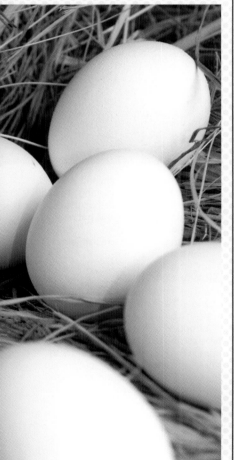

7 EAT REAL FOOD

This is key. Follow this rule and you'll end up following all the others almost by default. A simple rule of thumb is to eat only food that grew out of the ground or once had a face. Or go caveman and think like a hunter-gatherer. When looking at something on the shelf, ask yourself if it would have existed 5,000 years ago. If the answer's no, you probably shouldn't eat it.

You may find it easier to stick to the outer aisles of the supermarket, which is where the fresh produce is usually kept for ease of transportation, and away from the interior where everything's canned, processed or packed full of preservatives. Avoid things containing preservatives that you can't spell or ingredients you wouldn't keep in your kitchen cupboard. Eat things that will rot eventually so you know they're fresh. And try to enjoy it.

USING CARBS CORRECTLY

When building muscle and burning fat, using carbs can be one of the best ways to get ripped, as Nick Mitchell explains

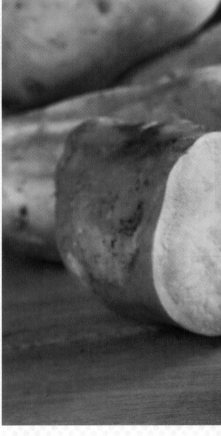

Carbohydrates have a pretty bad rap when it comes to muscle building and fat loss. They cause insulin levels to spike, which can result in your body storing more energy as fat rather than using fat for energy. But manipulating your carb intake is one of the best ways to get bigger and leaner. You just need to be lean enough in the first place to deserve those carbs.

Individual tolerance

At first glance, Joe's diet looks a lot like the dreaded Atkins diet. This isn't the case but you'll go a long way to understanding how to eat for fat loss if you can grasp that controlling your blood sugar is of paramount importance. This means carbs should only be introduced when and if your body can handle them properly.

The bad news is that if you're out of shape you can't handle them. The good news is that weight training and getting leaner and more muscular improves insulin sensitivity, so fewer of the carbs you ingest go into fat cells and go instead into muscle cells where we want them to go. This means that as the 12 weeks of the programme progress, you may in fact benefit from adding carbs into your diet at some point.

Joe is naturally tolerant of carbs, as is the case with most naturally skinny individuals. However, years of bad eating had hampered this ability to deal with them, so we needed to stick to a very low-carb diet for the initial weeks to get his body used to using fat as energy, rather than dietary carbohydrates, and to improve his insulin sensitivity that would in turn also make it easier to add muscle.

Carb cycling

After training hard and following a low-carb diet for two to six weeks, most individuals will benefit from selectively adding the right carbs into their diet. However, rather than simply eating carbs on a daily basis, science and anecdotal experience have shown that cycling your intake with low, medium and high-intake days will produce much better results for fat loss and muscle building.

This way you get the muscle-building benefit of high-carb days with the fat-loss benefits of lower-carb days, all while keeping your metabolism properly revved up with fluctuating daily calorie intakes.

One size doesn't fit all

Unfortunately, there's no one-size-fits-all approach to carb cycling. What worked in Joe's case may not work in yours, so it's important to read this part thoroughly to understand what you need to do. Pay very close attention to your body's feedback and adjust your intake according to the criteria we lay out for you below.

After adhering to my seven diet rules, explained above, for the first two weeks

'Manipulating your carb intake is one of the best ways to get bigger and leaner'

of the programme, you need to start reviewing your progress to determine when you need to reintroduce carbs. You'll know the time is right when you're eating sufficient quantities of the foods outlined in the diet but are beginning to suffer the following symptoms:

▶ You feel sluggish all the time.
▶ You're not getting a decent pump when you weight-train and your energy levels while training are generally much lower than usual.
▶ You normally sleep well but now your sleep is disturbed.
▶ You're noticeably more irritable than normal.

Slowly does it

If you are genuinely noticing these changes – and not just desperately craving a bagel – you need to reintroduce carbs slowly. When the time comes to add them to your diet, start in the first week by adding 50g of carbs to your post-workout shake. Joe used Poliquin Quadricarb but any fast-acting carb powder will do.

If this small addition of carbs helps to relieve the symptoms, the next step is to add a large bowl of porridge – made with water, not milk – before you go to bed on those days that you train. If you can't stomach porridge, you can substitute it

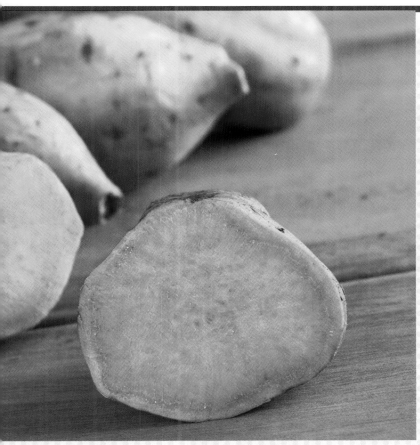

WHY SWEET POTATOES ARE OK
Slow-release carbs are the key to building muscle and burning fat

The glycaemic index is a scale from one to 100 that reveals how quickly a food affects your blood-sugar levels. The higher the number, the faster the energy gets into your bloodstream

and the quicker insulin levels rise. Slow-release carbs, such as sweet potatoes, release energy slowly so you don't get a sugar spike and crash, which can result in fat storage.

with a medium-size serving of wild rice, yams or sweet potatoes.

Aggressive tactics
If after two weeks of consuming these additional carbs you continue to feel better and are seeing yourself become leaner, this is the time to start thinking about more aggressive carb-cycling strategies.

Because we're interested in aggressive fat loss, for carb cycling to be effective you also need to manage your calorie intake. When you add

carbs, you must remove calories from that day's diet by reducing your protein and/or fat intake.

Before you freak out that eating less protein will result in a loss of your new muscles, don't worry – it won't, especially if you've been eating at the high end of the 4g per kilogram of bodyweight as I have advised. A good rule of thumb is if you add 100g of carbs to your diet, take away 50-100g of protein, but never let your protein intake fall below 2g per kilo of bodyweight.

5-DAY CARB CYCLING
Here's a five-day outline of how to effectively cycle your carb intake

Once you introduce carbs, most of your protein sources need to be white fish or turkey mince apart from at breakfast, which should be meat, preferably red, with nuts every day. The majority of carbs must come from porridge or sweet potatoes, but on high-carb days you can have one piece of fruit and one serving of low-fat dairy (milk or yoghurt) if you fancy them.

DAY ONE
Protein 250g
Carbs 50g post-workout/75g before bed

DAY TWO
Protein 300g (three servings of red meat)
Carbs 0g

DAY THREE
Protein 250g
Carbs 75g post-workout/150g over three servings after training

DAY FOUR
Protein 300g (three servings of red meat)
Carbs 0g

DAY FIVE
Protein 250g
Carbs 50g post-workout/75g before bed

WEEKLY MEAL PLAN

Now you know the food rules you need to stick to over the course of the 12-week challenge, you're armed with all the information you need to get started. However, if you are unsure of how all the rules fit together in your shopping trolley – rather than just on paper – here's a seven-day menu that is typical of the one Joe followed during his transformation.

Clear your cupboards
You're more likely to make bad food choices if you have tempting, unhealthy foods in your kitchen. Before you start the challenge, make sure you have a proper clear-out.

It's also worth throwing away any takeaway menus: you don't want to be reminded of what you need to avoid eating, and not having them at hand makes you less likely to give in to temptation.

Finally, stock up on all the foods and snacks that will be the staples of your diet for the next few months. And talk to your local butcher so you can be kept up-to-date on the best-quality stock he gets in.

MONDAY

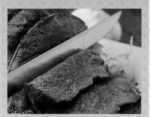

BREAKFAST
Roast beef slices with a handful of brazil nuts

MORNING SNACK
Two boiled eggs

PRE-WORKOUT
Beta-alanine shake with caffeine

POST-WORKOUT
Whey protein shake with creatine

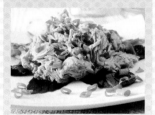

LUNCH
Tuna salad

AFTERNOON SNACK
Greek yoghurt

DINNER
Chicken breast with roasted vegetables

TUESDAY

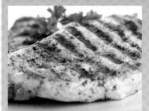

BREAKFAST
Chicken breast with a handful of almonds

MORNING SNACK
Protein shake

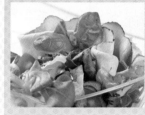

LUNCH
Ham salad

AFTERNOON SNACK
Raw vegetables with guacamole

DINNER
Steak with steamed green vegetables

WEDNESDAY

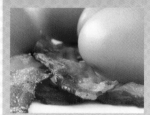

BREAKFAST
Bacon and two boiled eggs

MORNING SNACK
Tin of salmon

PRE-WORKOUT
Beta-alanine shake with caffeine

POST-WORKOUT
Whey protein shake with creatine

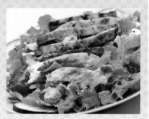

LUNCH
Turkey salad

AFTERNOON SNACK
Tin of tuna

DINNER
Cod fillet with steamed vegetables

THURSDAY	FRIDAY	SATURDAY	SUNDAY

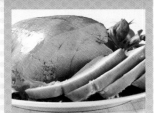

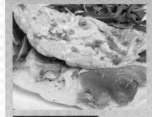

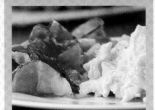

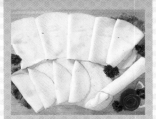

THURSDAY

BREAKFAST
Roast chicken slices with a handful of brazil nuts

MORNING SNACK
Two scrambled eggs

LUNCH
Chicken stir-fry

AFTERNOON SNACK
Raw vegetables with guacamole

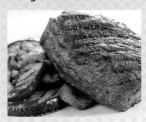

DINNER
Steak with roasted vegetables

FRIDAY

BREAKFAST
Ham omelette with a handful of almonds

MORNING SNACK
Tin of salmon

PRE-WORKOUT
Beta-alanine shake with caffeine

POST-WORKOUT
Whey protein shake with creatine

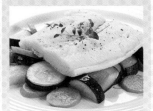

LUNCH
Cod fillet with steamed vegetables

AFTERNOON SNACK
Raw vegetables with guacamole

DINNER
Minced beef chilli with vegetables

SATURDAY

BREAKFAST
Bacon and two scrambled eggs

MORNING SNACK
Handful of almonds

PRE-WORKOUT
Beta-alanine shake with caffeine

POST-WORKOUT
Whey protein shake with creatine

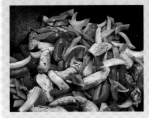

LUNCH
Chicken stir-fry

AFTERNOON SNACK
Tin of salmon

DINNER
Steak with roasted vegetables

SUNDAY

BREAKFAST
Turkey slices with a handful of brazil nuts

MORNING SNACK
Protein shake

LUNCH
Ham salad

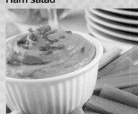

AFTERNOON SNACK
Raw vegetables with guacamole

DINNER
Roast beef with steamed vegetables

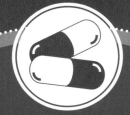

COMPLETE GUIDE TO SUPPLEMENTS

Read on to find out which pills and powders
can aid fat loss, boost muscle growth
and help you to recover faster

HELPING HAND

Take the right supplements to accelerate your progress

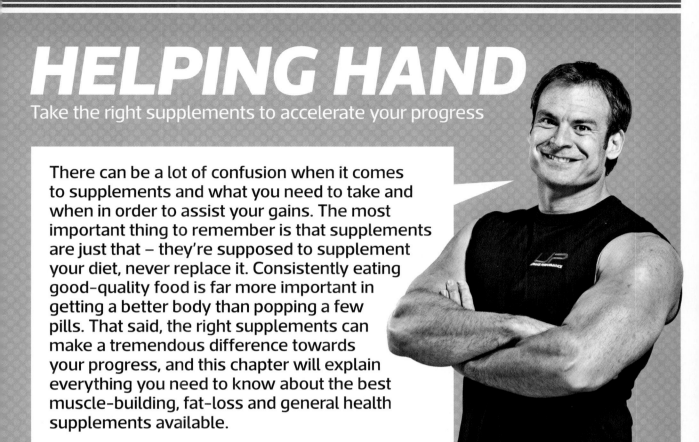

There can be a lot of confusion when it comes to supplements and what you need to take and when in order to assist your gains. The most important thing to remember is that supplements are just that – they're supposed to supplement your diet, never replace it. Consistently eating good-quality food is far more important in getting a better body than popping a few pills. That said, the right supplements can make a tremendous difference towards your progress, and this chapter will explain everything you need to know about the best muscle-building, fat-loss and general health supplements available.

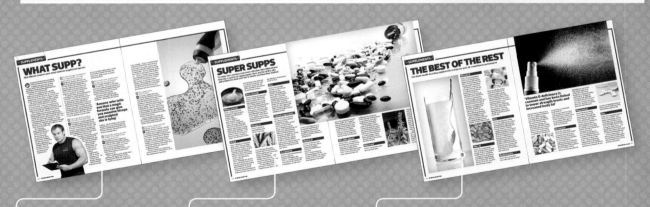

P160 When is the best time to take a supplement? And can they let you off a day in the gym? Nick answers these questions and more

P164 Learn which are the best supplements to take to fuel your muscle-building workouts and help torch unwanted fat

P166 These health-boosting supplements will mean you don't neglect the rest of your body while your working hard in the gym

WHAT SUPP?

Nick Mitchell answers your most common supplement queries

Supplements promise everything from torching your love handles to sculpting your pecs, but do they actually work? And which ones do you need? Our comprehensive guide tells you everything you need to know.

Whether you regularly pack a protein shake in your gym bag or sink an isotonic drink after sport, the chances are you've used supplements at one time or another. Trouble is, the whole process can get a bit confusing – with every supplier claiming its brand is better filtered, more efficient or will pack on more muscle – to the point where it can feel as if you need a degree in chemistry to understand what you're putting into your body.

Don't worry, help is at hand. The science may be baffling, but we've put together the definitive guide of the latest developments in supplement science: what you need, when you need it, why you need it and what – if any – are its potential pitfalls. It's possible you'll find something to send your training gains through the roof, or you might learn a bit more about what you're already using.

The following pages detail all the supplements Joe took on his cover model mission, followed by a round-up of the best muscle-building, fat-burning and general health supplements available. But first, Nick answers some of the most common questions about supplements.

Q If I take the right combination of supplements, can I get ripped without working out?

A Sadly, no. Anyone who tells you that a magic formula can give you massive biceps and sculpted abs is lying. Eat right, train hard, tailor your supplement use to your goals and choose well-researched and tested products, and you'll see results.

The point I make about supplements is that they're 'supplementary', not essentials. If you can afford them and you have your training and diet spot-on, then by all means experiment with them. Just remember, there is no substitute for correct eating and hard training, and that it's possible to make amazing progress just by sticking very much to the basics. Supplements are your icing on top of the cake when it comes to getting maximal results.

Q Can't I get all the nutrition I need from my daily diet?

A If you live on a tropical island with no pollution and naturally grown and reared food then possibly, yes. But if you live somewhere like the UK, with its mass-produced food (quantity not quality) and its polluted environment, then supplements have a huge role to play. Almost everyone, for example, should take a good-quality probiotic, fish oil and a multivitamin, just for basic good health. When trying to enhance body composition, we would look at performance-related supplements such as creatine. However, I always come from a position that we optimise health first before looking

at more esoteric supplements, simply because the healthier the body, the better your ability to put on muscle and burn body fat.

Q Do I need to take supplements on the days I'm not training?

A Yes. You get stronger as you recover from exercise, so making sure you're getting enough nutrients on your rest days is essential to keep your muscles fuelled and encourage fat stores to be used as energy.

Remember, the training in this programme stimulates an adaptive response – fat burning and muscle

'Anyone who tells you that a magic formula can give you massive biceps and sculpted abs is lying'

building – but it's what you do outside the gym when you're recovering that governs whether that stimulation has the raw materials and environment to produce the right effect.

Q Should I be waking up in the middle of the night to take certain supplements?

A Definitely not. You might have heard about bodybuilders getting up at 3am to neck a quick shake, but as soon as you're awake for more than three seconds you disrupt the production of melatonin, which is one of the most important hormones in building muscle.

Focus on getting good-quality sleep and leave the alarm clock for the morning only. What a lot of guys do – and this is a mistake I made when

I was younger – is have a protein shake waiting for them if they wake up to go to the toilet. I know this sounds rather innocuous and on the surface the logic is impeccable – if you're already awake, then why not get some extra nutrition in? – but it's a mistake because of the hormonal impact of food on 'breaking your fast'. Research has now shown that a seven- to ten-hour fasting window, which naturally occurs when we sleep, is fantastic for maximising growth-hormone production and promoting a lean and mean physique.

Q Are supplements safe to take?

A As sports supplements are technically classified as food, they aren't subject to the same strict manufacturing, safety testing or labelling as licensed medicines, so there's no guarantee they're living up to their claims. The EU is currently looking into the situation with a view to introducing stricter guidelines, but in the meantime it's up to individual manufacturers to maintain the quality of their own products.

Look for supplements that are ISO 17025 certified, which means they've been subjected to rigorous checks during their production.

Q Can I fail a drugs test after taking supplements?

A Maybe. If you're a serious enough sportsman to be tested, you must be cautious about supplements that may contain stimulants or prohormones. A survey by an International Olympic Committee-accredited laboratory in Cologne looked for steroids in 634 supplements and found 15% per cent contained substances that would cause a failed drug test, although none contained steroids.

If you're concerned, contact your sports federation and ask them about the supplement in question.

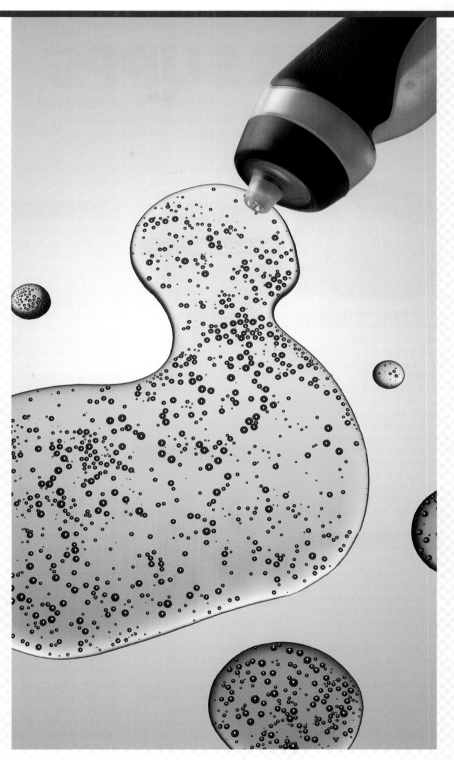

SUPER SUPPS

To make Joe's mission even more effective, Nick Mitchell had him take a variety of supplements. Here are the all the pills and potions he used over the 12 weeks and how they worked

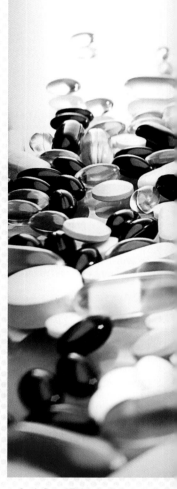

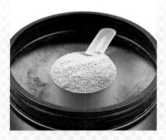

Whey protein

WHAT? A type of protein derived from dairy products, which is typically found in powder form.
WHEN? 50g in a post-workout shake.
WHY? Whey is digested quicker than any other type of protein, making it ideal to rapidly replenish your muscle tissues after training and kick-start protein synthesis, or the process where new muscle fibres are built, resulting in bigger and stronger muscles.

BCAA

WHAT? BCAAs, or branched-chain amino acids, are taken during heavy weight-training. Each capsule contains an ideal anabolic (muscle-building) ratio of the three amino acids, leucine, isoleucine and valine.
WHEN? 40-60g during every workout.
WHY? Taking BCAAs during your workout has numerous benefits, including preventing the breakdown of muscle tissue and post-workout soreness, and increasing post-workout muscle recovery and

testosterone levels. Nick had Joe take three capsules with water after every work set, which worked out at between 40 and 60 per session.

Beta-alanine

WHAT? A type of amino acid.
WHEN? About 30 minutes before training. Stick to the label guidelines for dosage.
WHY? This supplement is great for improving your levels of focus and concentration during your workouts. It also increases the concentration of the dipeptide carnosine in the muscle, which allows you to perform more reps during those intense weight-lifting sessions.

Omega 3

WHAT? A form of essential fatty acid.
WHEN? 5g a day.

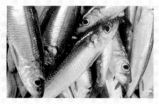

WHY? Omega 3 is mainly found in oily cold-water fish, such as salmon and anchovies, and is essential for good health. Research has shown it helps to prevent a host of long-term ailments, including cancer and heart disease.

It's especially beneficial when you're trying to lose weight because it promotes

the utilisation of existing fat stores for fuel.

Zinc

WHAT? An essential mineral we can only get through our diet.
WHEN? 10mg per day.
WHY? We need zinc for hundreds of essential biological functions, not least for the production of testosterone. However, despite this, many men have low levels. This supplement helps to restore adequate zinc levels for better muscle-building potential.

Topical magnesium

WHAT? A cream applied to the skin to restore optimal magnesium levels.
WHEN? Two squirts behind each knee before bed.
WHY? Magnesium is the fourth-most abundant mineral in the body and involved in 300 essential biochemical reactions, ranging from energy production in your cells to protein synthesis, making it vital for optimal athletic performance. Many people are deficient in magnesium and this cream can help to boost your levels.

L-carnitine

WHAT? A compound primarily found in red meat.
WHEN? 500mg per day.
WHY? L-carnitine plays many roles in the body, specifically in helping to use fat stores

as fuel. Carn-Enhanced is a convenient liquid form that also contains vitamins B5 and B12 to increase your fat-burning potential and improve energy levels.

Vitamin D

WHAT? A vitamin made by your body when skin is exposed to sunlight.
WHEN? 25,000IU twice per week.
WHY? A lack of regular, strong sunlight in the UK means most Brits are severely lacking in this crucial vitamin that supports bone health

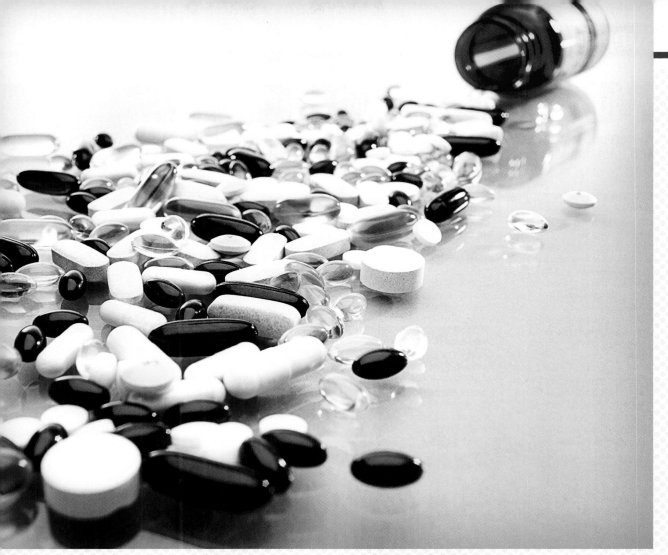

and a strong immune system. Many studies also suggest that vitamin D may decrease risk for many diseases and conditions, including certain types of cancer, multiple sclerosis and hypertension, as well as aid in weight loss and even improve longevity.

HCI with pepsin

WHAT? HCI is a compound that helps your body to break down the food you eat more efficiently and effectively.
WHEN? One tablet after meals.
WHY? If your stomach can't break down food into the building blocks of muscle, you're not only wasting money on good food, you're also wasting time in the gym.

Choose a form of the supplement that contains compounds that help you to extract vitamin B12 and iron from food, both of which are vital for good energy levels, as well as pepsin, herbal bitter and gentian root, all of which help to fire up your digestive system.

Holy basil

WHAT? An aromatic plant grown in the tropics.

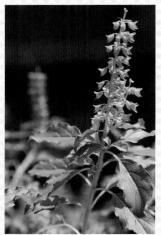

WHEN? Two tablets each with breakfast and lunch.
WHY? Compounds found in holy basil limit your cortisol response when you're faced with those daily disturbances that can make your blood boil. Having high levels of this stress hormone in your system is very damaging and can result in your body storing more fat around your belly.

Available in products such as Holy Basil Supreme, it can also protect the body from the effects of both physical and chemical stress and will boost your energy levels in the morning and afternoon.

MUSCLE UP

When you want to add lean muscle mass, these are the best supplements to help you reach your goals

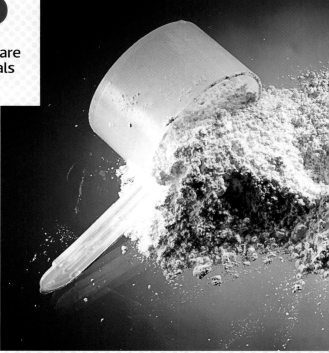

Whey protein

WHAT The post-workout protein

WHY Whey is a fast-release protein, which means it is quickly digested and so gets into your bloodstream – and therefore your muscles – fast. What you consume after training is one of the most important meals you eat, so make sure you buy a high-quality product.

HOW Your muscles are most receptive to nutrients as soon as you finish training, so drink a protein shake as soon as your final rep is completed. Aim for a minimum of 40g of whey protein powder.

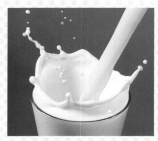

Casein

WHAT The bedtime protein

WHY Casein is a form of protein commonly found in dairy products – it makes up around 80% of cow's milk, for example. It's a slow-release protein because it takes longer for your body to digest, so you get more of a 'drip-feed' effect of protein into your bloodstream over a longer period. This makes it unsuitable for taking immediately after your

workout when you need an instant hit but ideal for consuming before bed.

HOW Have it in a shake with water before turning in for the night. This means your muscles will receive quality protein while you sleep, which is when they are repaired and rebuilt.

BCAA

WHAT The muscle pill

WHY Branched-chain amino acids are the best supplement to take during your workouts because they help to keep a steady supply of proteins flowing into your muscles. This has been proven to aid muscle building as it reduces the amount of muscle loss during exercise and improves protein synthesis, which is the process by which new muscle tissue is built. BCAAs can also help to prevent muscle loss during periods of intermittent fasting.

HOW Take up to 0.4g per kilogram of bodyweight during the course of your weight-training session.

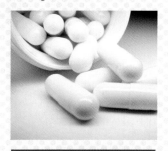

Creatine

WHAT The backup generator for your muscles

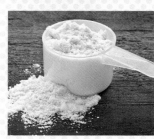

WHY Your body metabolises creatine into ATP, which is used for every initial muscle movement. It's therefore vital to have adequate supplies during heavy, high-intensity workouts to deliver the required energy to your muscles. In other words, creatine helps you lift harder for longer.

HOW Take 2-10g in your post-workout shake to replenish lost stores, or split your dose and have half before your workout and half after. And make sure you drink

plenty of water: creatine is hygroscopic, so it will suck water into your muscles and can leave you dehydrated.

Leucine

WHAT The muscle booster

WHY The most anabolic amino acid, leucine can independently stimulate insulin secretion and muscle protein synthesis, enhancing the muscle-building process. At 11%, whey protein is high in leucine content, which is one reason it's so effective as a post-workout elixir.

HOW A 5g dose of leucine after training and between meals can increase the anabolic – or muscle-building – effect of food, especially when consuming protein sources that are low in leucine and which therefore might not stimulate maximum muscle protein synthesis on their own.

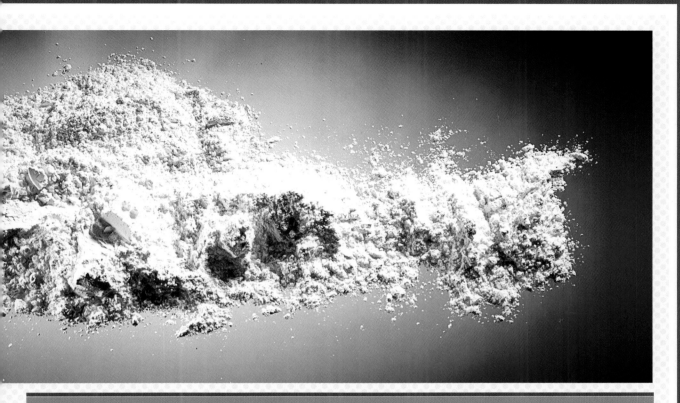

GET RIPPED

The most effective supplements for burning fat

Thermogenics

WHAT The metabolism booster

WHY Also known as fat burners, these mixtures of herbs and stimulants can increase your body temperature, helping you to torch fat. However, although they can work for a short-term boost, you should avoid long-term use.

HOW Stick to the label's guidelines when it comes to dose. You should avoid taking them after 2pm, however, because these stimulants may affect your sleep if taken any later in the day.

Green tea

WHAT The diet drink

WHY This is one of the best natural fat burners around and can give your metabolism a jolt. Green tea is also packed full of antioxidants and has been linked to the prevention of everything from heart disease to Alzheimer's.

HOW Drink instead of your regular tea or diet soft drink to reap a huge variety of health benefits.

Phosphatidyl serine

WHAT The cortisol buster

WHY Anyone training intensely is likely to be putting their body under some serious stress. In such situations the stress hormone cortisol, which is responsible for fat storage, is secreted in high amounts. However, phosphatidyl serine helps to block its secretion. This in turn allows you to recover quicker, burn more fat and build more muscle.

HOW Phosphatidyl serine can be taken at doses of 800mg after training or in the evening by those individuals who are prone to high stress or who are experiencing high training levels.

L-carnitine

WHAT The fat shredder

WHY If burning fat during a workout is your priority, first you need to mobilise it. L-carnitine is an amino acid responsible for transporting fatty acids into the mitochondria, our cells' energy powerhouses.

HOW Take a single dose of 500-3,000mg pre-workout to ensure you transport the maximum amount of available fat for fuel during exercise. It's especially useful if you're training while fasting or on a low-carb diet, when fat oxidation is maximised.

THE BEST OF THE REST

Use these health-boosting supplements to improve your all-round fitness performance

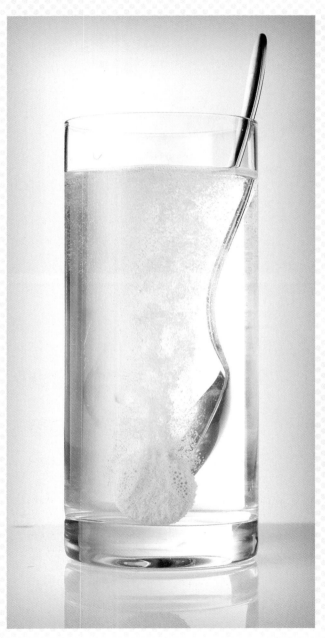

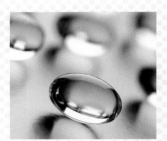

Vitamin D

WHAT The sun substitute
WHY You should get your vitamin D from the sun but that's a forlorn hope for the average deskbound Briton - 20 minutes' exposure is enough in the summer but according to the National Institute of Health, it's impossible to get enough come the winter. Deficiency is common and linked to lower strength levels and increased body fat. It has also been linked to a number of diseases, including cancer, diabetes and depression.
HOW It's available in tablet form or as an oral spray. Official government recommendations are low – aim for 3,000IU a day, which has been proved safe in multiple studies. It's fat-soluble, so take it with a meal.

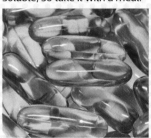

Fish oil

WHAT The wonder fluid
WHY It's important to include omega 3 fats in your diet for health reasons, and taking a supplement can help you to maintain a good omega 3 to omega 6 ratio. Modern humans, as a rule, consume far too much omega 6.

More specifically, studies have shown that fish oil supplementation results in decreased body fat and reduced inflammation. It has also been linked to increased serotonin levels, more focus in training and less stress.
HOW Take a spoonful with your meals. Most authorities recommend 1-4g a day, depending on how much oily fish is already included in your diet.

HCL

WHAT The digestion helper
WHY HCL (hydrochloric acid) is responsible for digesting and breaking down animal protein in your stomach. Taking a supplement will ensure you're actually getting the benefit of all the protein you're eating. If you aren't digesting and breaking down nutrients properly in your gut, then all other supplements and healthy food could simply be wasted as you won't be able to absorb them effectively.
HOW Take one or two tablets with each meal.

Multivitamins

WHAT The backup plan
WHY Although you shouldn't

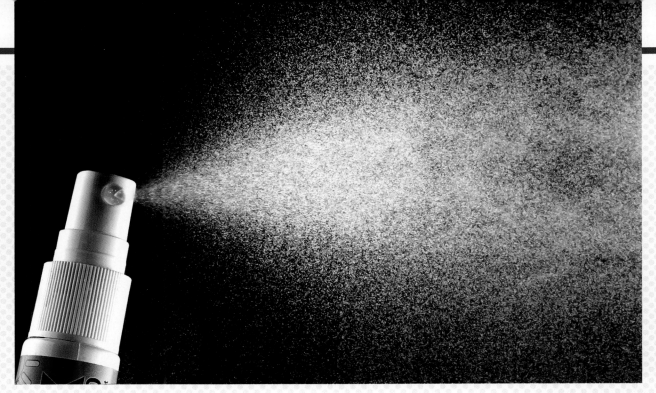

'Vitamin D deficiency is common and has been linked to lower strength levels and increased body fat'

rely on them to make up for a bad diet, a quality multivitamin can help to fill in the gaps in an otherwise solid eating plan. Deficiencies in vitamins can cause mood swings, depression, lethargy and exhaustion but taking a daily dose will keep you on the up and focused on your goals. There is also evidence that a multivitamin can help you

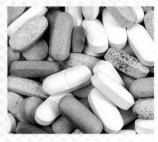

recover from a particularly tough workout.

HOW You should aim to take multivitamins at a consistent time of the day. It makes sense to take them before a meal, for example, with a glass of water to aid absorption of their micronutrients.

Glutamine

WHAT The gut calmer
WHY This amino acid should already be present in your body. However, if you have problems with your digestion or are training hard, a supplement can be helpful to strengthen the lining of your gut and help protein synthesis.
HOW You have several options on how you take this,

depending on your goals. Take 10g in water on an empty stomach before breakfast to aid in gut healing and function, or 10g post-workout to help replenish your glutamine store. If you're on a low-carb diet, take 30g after your workout to enhance glycogen replenishment.

Magnesium

WHAT The body calmer
WHY Every organ needs magnesium, especially the heart, muscles and kidneys. If you skimp on this vital mineral you can experience anxiety, sleep problems and irritability. It also helps to maintain a normal heart rhythm and aids in the body's energy production.
HOW You should stick to the recommended dose of less than 350mg a day and remember to take it with food – taking magnesium supplements on an empty stomach can lead to diarrhoea and an upset stomach. Or you

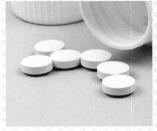

can use a magnesium spray or lotion, both of which are easily absorbed through the skin.

Zinc

WHAT The masculine mineral
WHY Zinc is vital for your health and immune system. Our bodies can't store it, so you need to top up regularly.
HOW The RDA intake for zinc is 11mg for adult males – you should take no more than 40mg. Don't take it with coffee or foods containing phytates – such as wholegrains – as they can block its absorption. For the best benefits, take it with animal proteins as they promote absorption.

TRAINING DIARY

This simple workout planner allows you follow the 12-week training programme with ease and record all the weights you lift for every move, so it's easy to chart your progress

STAY ON TRACK

Use this training diary to chart your progress

The only way to get the most out of every session is to know exactly what you need to do as soon as you get in the gym. That's why a training diary is so important. All the exercises, sets, reps, tempo and rests are clearly detailed in each chapter, but the one thing that's unique to you is the weight you need to lift. That's where this training log comes in. Simply note down the weight you used to successfully complete all the sets and reps and the desired tempo. Then you'll know what increase you need to make next time to keep your muscles growing and avoid a dreaded growth plateau.

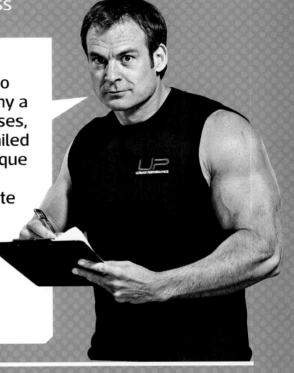

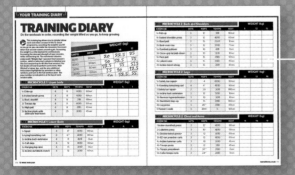

P170 Our simple-to-follow training log will help you keep track of the weights you're lifting in each session. Just don't forget your pencil!

KEEPING TRACK

Do the workouts in order and record the weight lifted as you go to keep growing

This training log allows you to record the weight you lift in each and every session in this 12-week programme as you go, so you can keep track of your progress and, if necessary, make increases when that session comes around again. Increasing the weight is a vital element in continuously increasing the size and strength of your muscles, while still burning fat.

The numbered columns underneath 'Weight (kg)' represent that session's number, which is why each column is labelled from 1 (the first session) to 46 (the final session). For full details of how to perform each move, Nick Mitchell's trainer tips and for any additional instructions highlighted by asterisks or other symbols, just turn to the full workout plan. The page number is indicated at the top of each session table.

TEMPO	REST	WEIGHT (kg) 11	14	17
4010	90sec	20	22.5	25
4010	90sec	50	52.5	55
3010	60sec	52.5	55	57.5
4010	60sec	7.5	10	12.5
		50	52.5	55

P38 MICROCYCLE 1 Upper body

EXERCISE	SETS	REPS	TEMPO	REST	WEIGHT (kg) 1	3	5	7
1a Chin-up	4	8	4010	90sec				
1b Incline bench press	4	8	4010	90sec				
2a Rack deadlift	4	8	2111	90sec				
2b Triceps dip	4	8	4010	90sec				
3a High pull	4	8	2110	45sec				
3b Decline plank with alternate foot touch	4	25	2010	45sec				

P42 MICROCYCLE 1 Lower body

EXERCISE	SETS	REPS	TEMPO	REST	WEIGHT (kg) 2	4	6	8
1a Squat	4	8*	4010	90sec				
1b Lying hamstring curl	6	6**	4010	90sec				
2a Incline back extension	4	8	4011	0sec				
2b Calf raise	4	12	4010	90sec				
3a Hanging leg raise	4	15	3010	0sec				
3b Decline dumbbell crunch	4	12	3010	90sec				

P46 MICROCYCLE 2 Back and shoulders

EXERCISE	SETS	REPS	TEMPO	REST	WEIGHT (kg) 9	12	15
1a Pull-up	3	12	3111	60sec			
1b Seated shoulder press	3	12	4010	60sec			
2a Band pull	3	15	20X1	10sec			
2b Bent-over row	3	12	3010	75sec			
3a Dumbbell pull-over	3	10	4111	0sec			
3b Close-grip lat pull-down	3	10	3011	10sec			
3c Face pull	3	15	2010	90sec			
4a Lateral raise	3	15	2010	45sec			
4b Incline bench shrug	3	15	2011	45sec			

P50 MICROCYCLE 2 Legs

EXERCISE	SETS	REPS	TEMPO	REST	WEIGHT (kg) 10	13	16
1a Safety bar squat+	2	4	6010	90sec			
1b Kneeling hamstring curl	4	4*	4010	90sec			
2 Safety bar squat+	2	20	3011	180sec			
3a Incline back extension	3	12	3012	10sec			
3b Reverse hyperextension	3	10	3011	10sec			
4a Dumbbell step-up	3	15	2010	180sec			
4b Leg press	3	45**	2010	60sec			
5 Farmer's walk	3	40m	X	90sec			

P54 MICROCYCLE 2 Chest and arms

EXERCISE	SETS	REPS	TEMPO	REST	WEIGHT (kg) 11	14	17
1 Incline dumbbell bench press	3	12*	4010	90sec			
2 Guillotine press	3	10*	4010	90sec			
3a Decline bench press+	3	12	3010	60sec			
3b EZ-bar preacher curl	3	12	4010	60sec			
4a Incline hammer curl	3	10	3010	45sec			
4b Triceps press	3	12	3110	45sec			
5a Triceps pressdown	2	30**	2010	0sec			
5b Cable biceps curl	2	24**	2010	0sec			

P60 MICROCYCLE 3 Back and shoulders — WEIGHT (kg) 18

EXERCISE	SETS	REPS	TEMPO	REST	
1 Underhand lat pull-down	2	10	4010	60sec	
2 Seated cable row	2	10*	3010	60sec	
3 Reverse bench row	1	10*	3010	90sec	
4 Seated dumbbell shoulder press	1	15	3010	90sec	
5 Cable lateral raise	2	12*	3010	60sec	
6 Face pull	2	12*	3010	60sec	

P63 MICROCYCLE 3 Legs — WEIGHT (kg) 19

EXERCISE	SETS	REPS	TEMPO	REST	
1a Lying hamstring curl	2	6*	4010	30sec	
1b Squat	2	12**	3010	60sec	
2 Leg press	1	50	1010	120sec	
3a Farmer's walk	4	40m	X	0sec	
3b Reverse sled drag	4	40m	X	90-120sec	
4a Decline plank with foot touch	4	24	2111	30sec	
4b Garhammer raise	4	12	2010	60sec	

P66 MICROCYCLE 3 Chest and arms — WEIGHT (kg) 20

EXERCISE	SETS	REPS	TEMPO	REST	
1 Incline dumbbell bench press	2	10	3010	90sec	
2 Incline dumbbell flye	2	12	3010	90sec	
3 Pectoral dip	1	F*	4010	90sec	
4a Spider curl	2	12	3011	60sec	
4b Decline EZ-bar triceps extension	2	12	4010	60sec	
5a Standing cable hammer curl	2	12**	3010	60sec	
5b Incline EZ-bar triceps press	2	12+	4010	60sec	
6 Diamond press-up	1	F*	3010	0sec	

P72 MICROCYCLE 4 Back and shoulders

EXERCISE	SETS	REPS	TEMPO	REST	WEIGHT (kg)		
					21	24	27
1a Rack deadlift	5	5	3111	90sec			
1b Seated dumbbell shoulder press	5	5	4010	90sec			
2a Reverse incline dumbbell row	4	6	3010	90sec			
2b Dumbbell high pull	4	6	2010	90sec			
3a Incline reverse lateral raise	3	15	3010	0sec			
3b Dumbbell shrug	3	15	2010	0sec			
3c Face pull	3	15	2010	60sec			

P76 MICROCYCLE 4 Legs

EXERCISE	SETS	REPS	TEMPO	REST	WEIGHT (kg)		
					22	25	28
1a Squat	6	6*	4010	150sec			
1b Lying hamstring curl	6	4*	4011	120sec			
2a Reverse sled drag	4	40m	X	0sec			
2b Dumbbell step-up	4	15	2010	90sec			

P78 MICROCYCLE 4 Chest and arms

EXERCISE	SETS	REPS	TEMPO	REST	WEIGHT (kg)		
					23	26	29
1a Incline bench press	5	5	4010	90sec			
1b Chin-up	5	5	4010	90sec			
2a Triceps dip	4	7	3010	75sec			
2b Preacher dumbbell hammer curl	4	7	3010	75sec			
3a Barbell rollout	4	6	4010	60sec			
3b Hanging leg raise	4	12	4010	90sec			

P84 MICROCYCLE 5 Back and shoulders

EXERCISE	SETS	REPS	TEMPO	REST	WEIGHT (kg) 30	33	36
1a Pull-up	3	6	4010	10sec			
1b Dumbbell pull-over	3	8	3010	10sec			
1c Seated cable row	3	8	3010	10sec			
1d Rack deadlift	3	10	2111	120sec			
2a Seated shoulder press	3	6	4010	0sec			
2b Cable lateral raise	3	10	2010	0sec			
2c Cable upright row	3	12	2010	90sec			

P88 MICROCYCLE 5 Legs

EXERCISE	SETS	REPS	TEMPO	REST	WEIGHT (kg) 31	34	37
1a Lying hamstring curl	4	6	3010	10sec			
1b Weighted glute bridge	4	10	2011	0sec			
1c Walking dumbbell lunge	4	40m	x	90sec			
2a Front squat*	10	6	3010	0sec			
2b Squat	10	9	3010	60sec			
3a Barbell rollout	4	6	4010	0sec			
3b Hanging leg raise	4	12	4010	30sec			
3c Decline dumbbell crunch	4	12	2010	60sec			

P92 MICROCYCLE 5 Chest and arms

EXERCISE	SETS	REPS	TEMPO	REST	WEIGHT (kg) 32	35	38
1a Incline dumbbell bench press	3	6	3110	10sec			
1b Decline bench press	3	6	4010	10sec			
1c Dumbbell bench press	3	6	4010	90sec			
2a EZ-bar preacher curl	3	6	4010	10sec			
2b Incline dumbbell curl	3	6	3110	10sec			
2c Kneeling overhead cable curl	3	6	3011	10sec			
2d Triceps dip	3	6	4010	10sec			
2e Decline lying triceps extension	3	6	4010	10sec			
2f Standing overhead triceps extension	3	6	3110	45sec			

P100 MICROCYCLE 6 Back and shoulders

EXERCISE	SETS	REPS	TEMPO	REST	WEIGHT (kg) 39
1a Lat pull-down	2	10	4010	90sec	
1b Seated cable row	2	10*	3010	90sec	
2a Reverse bench row	1	10*	3010	0sec	
2b Seated dumbbell shoulder press	1	15	3010	30sec	
3a Cable lateral raise	2	12*	3010	0sec	
3b Face pull	2	12*	3010	30sec	
4 Barbell rollout	3	8	4010	60sec	

P104 MICROCYCLE 6 Legs

EXERCISE	SETS	REPS	TEMPO	REST	WEIGHT (kg) 40
1a Lying hamstring curl	2	6*	4010	90sec	
1b Squat	2	12*	3010	120sec	
2 Leg press	1	50	1010	180sec	
3a Farmer's walk	4	30m	X	0sec	
3b Reverse sled drag	4	30m	X	180sec	
4a Decline dumbbell crunch	4	12	3010	30sec	
4b Toes to bar	4	10	3010	0sec	
4c Hanging leg raise	4	10	3010	60sec	

P108 MICROCYCLE 6 Chest and arms

EXERCISE	SETS	REPS	TEMPO	REST	WEIGHT (kg) 41
1a Incline bench press	2	10	3010	30sec	
1b Incline dumbbell flye	2	12	3010	30sec	
2 Triceps dip	1	F*	4010	90sec	
3a Spider curl	2	12	3011	0sec	
3b Decline EZ-bar triceps extension+	2	12	4010	90sec	
4a Standing cable hammer curl	2	12*	3010	0sec	
4b Incline EZ-bar triceps press	2	12	4010	0sec	
5 Diamond press-up	1	F**	2010	90sec	

P114 MICROCYCLE 7 Back and shoulders — WEIGHT (kg) 42

EXERCISE	SETS	REPS	TEMPO	REST	
1a Pull-up	3	8	4010	10sec	
1b Dumbbell pull-over	3	10	3111	0sec	
1c Seated cable row	3	12	3010	90sec	
2a Reverse bench row	3	12	3011	0sec	
2b Seated dumbbell shoulder press	3	10	4010	90sec	
3a Incline reverse dumbbell flye	3	20	2010	0sec	
3b Face pull	3	20	2010	90sec	

P118 MICROCYCLE 7 Legs — WEIGHT (kg) 43

EXERCISE	SETS	REPS	TEMPO	REST	
1 Squat	5	12	4010	60sec	
2a Walking dumbbell lunge	5	70m	X	120sec	
2b Reverse sled drag	5	70m	x	180sec	
3 Calf raise	4	15	2010	90sec	

P120 MICROCYCLE 7 Chest and arms — WEIGHT (kg) 44

EXERCISE	SETS	REPS	TEMPO	REST	
1 Incline dumbbell bench press	3	10	4010	90sec	
2a Incline dumbbell flye	3	10	3110	0sec	
2b Triceps dip	3	10	4010	90sec	
3a Incline dumbbell curl	3	10	3111	0sec	
3b Decline EZ-bar triceps press	3	12	4010	90sec	
4a EZ-bar decline preacher curl	3	10	3010	0sec	
4b Standing overhead triceps extension	3	10	3010	90sec	

P126 MICROCYCLE 8 Legs and arms

EXERCISE	SETS	REPS	TEMPO	REST	WEIGHT (kg) 45
1a Walking dumbbell lunge	5	40m	2010	0sec	
1b Hex bar deadlift	5	20	2010	0sec	
1c Lying hamstring curl	5	10	2011	0sec	
1d Sissy squat	5	15	2010	120sec	
2a Incline dumbbell curl	4	15	2010	0sec	
2b Decline EZ-bar triceps press	4	15	2010	0sec	
2c Incline hammer curl	4	15	2011	0sec	
2d Decline EZ-bar triceps extension	4	15	2010	90sec	

P130 MICROCYCLE 8 Chest, back and shoulders

EXERCISE	SETS	REPS	TEMPO	REST	WEIGHT (kg) 46
1a Chin-up	3	12	2010	0sec	
1b Triceps dip	3	15	2010	75sec	
2a Reverse bench row	3	12	2010	0sec	
2b Incline dumbbell bench press	3	12	2010	75sec	
3a Seated cable row	3	15	3010	0sec	
3b Dumbbell bench press	3	15	3010	75sec	
4a Face pull	3	15	2011	0sec	
4b Cable crossover	3	25	3011	60sec	

Try 3 issues for just £1 and get the body you've always wanted!

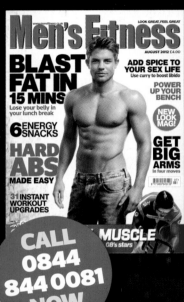

CALL 0844 844 0081 NOW

Inside Men's Fitness

New workouts to help you build muscle

Meal plans that strip away fat

Fitness advice from leading experts

Winning tips from top sportsmen

Gear for active men tested and rated

Plus you can add digital access for just 67p more per issue

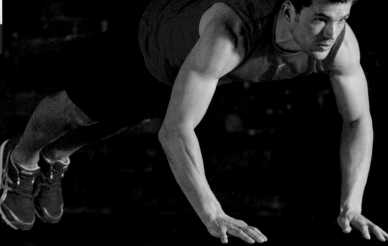

Claim 3 issues of *Men's Fitness* for £1!

Order online today at www.dennismags.co.uk/mensfitness

CALL 0844 844 0081

quoting code G1201BMB for print + digital or G1201PMB for print only

If during your 3 issues, you decide Men's Fitness isn't for you, simply cancel and you won't pay a penny more. But if you continue reading you'll SAVE 16% on the shop price, and pay just £19.95 every 6 issues.